"This book makes a unique, spirited push toward providing solace and education for young patients. In **Is My Brain Broken?** Dr. Deborah Lee provides first-person testimonials of children suffering from neurological diseases."

–**Clarion Review**

"A doctor explains neurological diseases in language easily understood by affected children. A compassionate project that informs and encourages young minds grappling with the fact that their brains may work differently from others."

–**Kirkus Reviews**

Is My Brain Broken?

Is My Brain Broken?

A Manual on Disorders of the Nervous System
Written for Kids by Kids

A Collection of Essays Written by Children Sharing Their Experiences
and Insights on Living and Coping with Neurological Disorders

Deborah Lee, MD, PhD
Pediatric Neurologist

Copyright © 2015 by Deborah Lee, MD, PhD.

Library of Congress Control Number: 2015912213
ISBN: Hardcover   978-1-5035-9101-1
              Softcover   978-1-5035-9102-8
              eBook   978-1-5035-9100-4

All rights reserved. No part of this book may be reproduced or transmitted in any form or by any means, electronic or mechanical, including photocopying, recording, or by any information storage and retrieval system, without permission in writing from the copyright owner.

Any people depicted in stock imagery provided by Thinkstock are models, and such images are being used for illustrative purposes only.
Certain stock imagery © Thinkstock.

Print information available on the last page.

Rev. date: 11/16/2015

To order additional copies of this book, contact:
Xlibris
1-888-795-4274
www.Xlibris.com
Orders@Xlibris.com
625959

and

Chance (age 7)

Steven (age 16)

Ashlyn (age 14)

Laura (age 11)

Kirkland (age 16)

Caine (age 7)

Geniece (age 11)

Claudia (age 11)

Keri (age 9)

Christopher (age 15)

Aaron (age 13)

Brittani (age 13)

Spencer (age 9)

Robert (age 10)

Megan (age 10)

Shanda (age 13)

Ryan (age 10)

Tyler (age 7)

Maddie (age 11)

Ashley (age 12)

Lana (age 7)

ACKNOWLEDGMENTS

First, I would like thank not only the children that participated in this book but also the children I had the privilege of caring for while I was in practice. I believe that they taught me more about their diseases than textbooks ever could. It is really their courage that has inspired me in my own life. In addition to providing the initial essays, fourteen years later, they have provided updates on how well they have done.

I especially want to thank our artists who provided, along with their stories, some very impressive art. Lana, aged seven years, who has two siblings with seizures, expressed her confusion on why her brother and sister have seizures but she and her other sister do not. She was given the opportunity to participate in the Studio E: Epilepsy Art Therapy Program for children with epilepsy and their siblings. So I would like to thank Lana, Studio E, and Epilepsy Foundation of Greater Cincinnati and Columbus for providing the striking cover art. I would also like to thank Maddie, aged eleven years, for providing all the internal art. Maddie has ADD but, much to her parents' surprise, sat for periods of three hours concentrating on her drawings. She was provided only the words in this book, and the pictures she drew were all her own. I would also like to thank her mother, Rachel, for her copy-editing skills.

I would also like to thank my husband, Dr. Craig Zwizinski, who has completely supported me throughout my career, and I do appreciate all the sacrifices he has made along the way.

Finally, I would like to thank my parents, Charles and Dorothy Lee, who raised me to believe I could do whatever I wanted to do and be whatever I wanted to be. And to especially thank my father, who gave me the courage to pursue my dream of publishing this book by publishing four of his own.

Contents

Preface — xiii

General Introduction — xvii

    An Overview of How the Nervous System Works

The Disorders — 1

    Common Nervous System Problems — 3

        Seizures and Epilepsy — 5

        Headaches — 31

            Migraines, Tension Headaches, Chronic Daily Headaches

    Nervous System Problems That Can Affect Behavior — 55

        ADHD/ADD — 57

        Autism — 69

    Nervous System Problems That Affect Strength — 107

        Weakness — 109

            Myopathies, Neuropathies

        Cerebral Palsy — 127

Nervous System Problems That Affect Movement	**133**
Tics and Tourette's Syndrome	135
More Movement Disorders	141
Friedreich's Ataxia, Parkinson's Disease	
Other Nervous System Problems	**171**
Autoimmune Disease	173
Guillain-Barré Syndrome, Transverse Myelitis, Multiple Sclerosis	
Brain Tumors	192
Final Lessons	**207**
Conclusion	**209**
Resources	**211**
Index	**215**

PREFACE

(For Adults)

WHY ANOTHER BOOK about disorders of the nervous system in children? There are certainly many good resources available for the general public, and some of the books have included essays by patients. However, even in these cases, contributions by the parents often took precedence, and the explanatory text was written for adults.

This book was written for children and, for the most part, by children. Kids do want to know what is wrong with them. These essays are presented exactly as the kids wrote them. There is significant variability between the essays written by the children, which reflects the age range of contributors (aged seven through sixteen) as well as the differential impact of their underlying neurological disease.

Descriptions and explanations are at a level that a child can understand. The book does not go into great detail about each subject, and certainly, adults and older children who want more information are encouraged to seek out more advanced texts. Few contributions by parents were solicited. This was a deliberate decision, as I wanted nothing to distract from the words of the children themselves. I was surprised at how often they commented that they wanted the doctors to talk to them; I was also distressed to hear how often they felt they were excluded. However, I hope that both children and their parents will read this book together. And although written for children, I anticipate that adults will also find the book illuminating. To this end, I have concluded most chapters with a section entitled "Lessons for Adults." Here, I will summarize what the children want us to understand about their disease and how we may better serve them.

Unlike the previous books, which have focused on a single disease, the topics included here cover a broad range. There is a chapter on one of the most common complaints of childhood (headaches); chapters on relatively common neurologic problems such as seizures, ADHD, and tics; and then finally, a few chapters discussing some of the more unusual manifestations of nervous system dysfunction such as brain tumors and diseases of the muscles and nerves. Again, this choice was deliberate. There is a high incidence of coexistence among these disorders, and children struggling with seizures often will also have to deal with migraines. Kids with ADHD may manifest tics, either as a related disorder or because of the side effects of the medication, and over a quarter of the patients with autism or cerebral palsy will have seizures. Therefore, I thought it would be useful to have one book that covered many topics, since most kids may have more than one diagnosis.

In addition, I hope that this book will be useful in a hospital setting so that families facing a new and frightening illness would have a child-friendly guide to help provide answers in an easily understood format. In addition, teachers, scout leaders, day-care workers, medical-care professionals, classmates, friends, and neighbors should be encouraged to learn more about these conditions. No adult needs to be an expert on seizures, but all adults in any kind of supervisory capacity should know what to do if a child under their care has one. Finally, it is important to include the siblings in these discussions as they are often confused about what is happening in the family.

Throughout the book, I have employed many metaphors to help children (and their parents) understand what is happening to them and why. These are not meant to be taken literally and are not always correlated with exact physiological mechanisms, most of which are not completely understood. I have found them very useful in helping a child cope with the question, "What is wrong with me?" However, some younger children might find them frightening; therefore, again, I would strongly recommend that this book be read by the child with the parent who can allay any fears the child might express.

In many essays, it is quite clear that the children gain much comfort from their spiritual beliefs. We do not, in any way, mean to encourage one set of beliefs over another. However, children often find strength in the idea that there is Someone, more powerful than they are, who cares for them and gives meaning to their lives.

The stories themselves are inspiring. For example, a child with two brain tumors teaches us how to truly value what we have been given instead of agonizing over what we lack. I am struck by the fact that not one of these children asked "Why me?" or sought to lay blame.

Finally, the true strength of this book lies with the updates provided by the children—now adults, fourteen years later. Here, they demonstrate that no matter the diagnosis they received as children, nothing has stopped them from succeeding in life. However, some of the follow-up essays describe some difficult choices that these children have had to make, and parents might want to read these sections beforehand. But the greatest lesson is that they are proud of their accomplishments no matter how difficult life has been.

GENERAL INTRODUCTION

How Does My Brain Really Work?

What Is the Brain?

THE BRAIN IS your body's central computer and controls everything your body does, including all your thinking and feeling. There are three major parts to your brain that you can see outlined in the picture below.

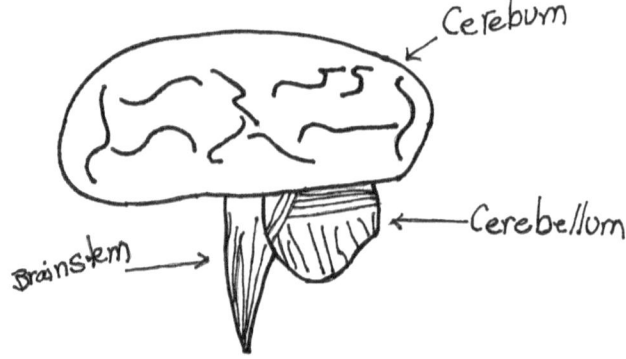

The first part, which is at the bottom, is called the brain stem. This part makes sure that you breathe and your heart beats, and the best part is that you don't even have to think about it. Another important part is called the cerebellum. This part makes sure that everything gets done at the right time. Finally, the last part, the one on top, is the cerebrum. This is the area of the brain that you think with and stores all your memories. This is also the part of the brain that lets you feel happy, sad, or angry.

The whole brain is protected by the hard skull and by layers of fluid (which looks like water) between the brain and the bone. These layers of fluid, as well as little pillows of fluid in the center of the brain, help protect the brain from getting hurt.

The brain talks to itself and the rest of your body by using both chemicals and electricity. The chemicals are very special and made by the brain. There are many different chemicals, and each one carries a different message. For example, one chemical might tell the brain (and you) to wake up, and another might tell the brain (and you) to go to sleep. So you can see that there can be big problems if you have too much of one chemical and not enough of another. One of the chemicals is almost the same as the chemical that your body makes when you are worried about something or frightened or even excited (like during finals or an important baseball game). Now you can understand why the brain (and you) may act funny when you are really upset.

The brain also uses electricity. Since it is the central computer, it has to send important information down long wires that run throughout your body (sort of like the electric cord that runs from the lamp to the wall). The wires are called nerves and are covered with something called insulation (like the rubbery stuff on the outside of the electric cord). This insulation keeps the electricity from escaping from the wires. These wires go all throughout your body so that every part of your body is under the brain's control. Some of the wires go the other way, and these wires bring information back to the brain. The nerves use both electricity *and* chemicals to carry messages!

An example of how the nervous system works would be what happens if you accidentally put your hand on something hot. The wires from your fingers to your brain carry the message "hot" to the brain. The brain decodes this message using those special chemicals (think of it like the brain's version of a secret-decoder ring!) into "ouch!" and realizes that something bad is happening. The brain then sends signals back down wires that tell the muscles to move the hand. The cerebellum watches over everything to make sure that the hand moves in the right direction, which is away from the hot object. And the best part is that the brain takes care of all this without you having to think about it!

The brain and nerves make up what we call the nervous system. Even though the muscles are a separate organ, they are often included because they work very closely with the nerves.

Why Is My Brain Like It Is?

Everybody's brain is different. We all like different things, have different skills and abilities, and have different personalities. Some people's brains are better at math and science, others at art, and others at sports. What determines what your brain will be like? Well, think of your brain as a giant jigsaw puzzle. Many different pieces go into making up your brain. The biggest piece will come from your parents.

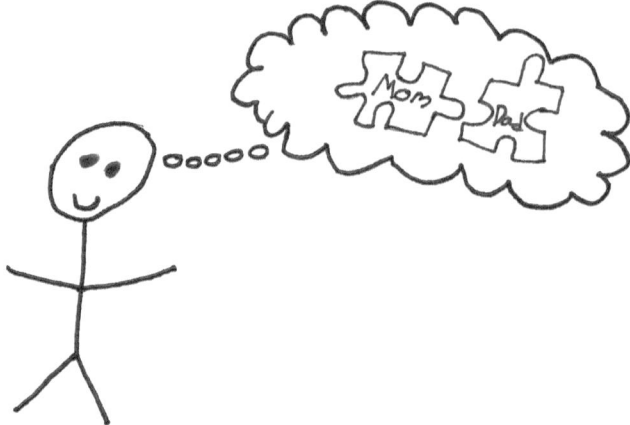

There are things called genes that carry all the information from your parents to make up *you*. Your brain often tends to turn out a lot like theirs. We call this heredity. Another important piece is how your brain grows before you are born. This is known as development. Finally, things that happen to your brain after you are born can also have a big effect. For example, if you injure your brain in an accident, the brain may have real problems carrying out its job (which is why we really want you to wear helmets when you ride your bicycle, scooter, or rollerblades)! The important thing to remember is that everybody's brains are good at doing some things and bad at doing other things.

What Happens When Things Go Wrong?

Just like any other part of your body, the brain can get sick too. When that happens, it can be pretty frightening. When the brain is sick or hurt, it can make you do all sorts of funny, scary, and uncool things. When you have a problem with your brain, you go to a special brain doctor (neurologist), who can help you find out what is wrong. Does your brain have an infection? Or did one part get hurt? Did it run out of blood (blood is very important to the brain because blood carries food to the brain), or is there a tumor? Sometimes we can't figure out why a brain has problems, especially if the problems have been there since birth.

Imagine a house with crooked windows and sagging floors. Is the house like this because the guy who drew the plans made a mistake (heredity)? Or did that guy do a great job, but the builders didn't know how to follow the plans (development)? Or finally, was the house built perfectly but got hit by a hurricane or burned down (an accident)? Many times, the doctors can figure out what is wrong and fix the problem. But sometimes, even if we can figure out what is wrong, it can't be fixed. This means you may have to get used to having a different brain from before, one which will now work in a different way. But don't worry–there are a lot of people who can help you! Like with the brain, problems can occur in the nerves and muscles. Like with the brain, some of those problems can be fixed and some can't.

How Does the Doctor Examine Your Brain?

There are many tests that a doctor can do to figure out what is wrong with your brain, nerves, or muscles. To see what the brain looks like, he or she may take a picture. A CT scan (computerized axial tomography) machine looks like a noisy giant doughnut, and an MRI (magnetic resonance imaging) machine looks like a noisy giant tunnel. Below is a picture of someone in an MRI.

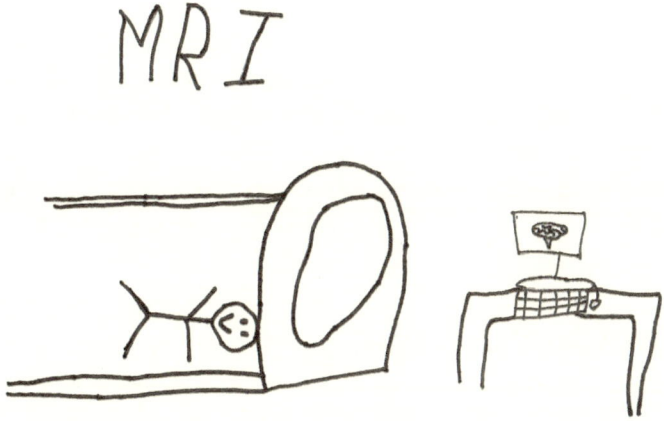

The MRI is a magnet, so you can't wear any metal during this test or you will stick to the machine. Both of these kinds of pictures can help the doctor look for anything wrong, like tumors.

Sometimes doctors will want to see how the electricity in the brain, nerves, or muscles is working. To see if the electricity in your brain is doing its job, they will order an EEG. An EEG measures your brain's electricity by hooking you up to special wires attached to a machine. The electrical power in your brain sends a signal that the machine can read, and doctors can tell from these signals if the electricity in your brain is working okay. They can use this machine to look for tiny electrical storms that might mean a person is having seizures (big electrical storms).

Sometimes we have to examine the muscles and the nerves. We can measure how fast and how many wires are carrying electricity down your nerves to your muscles (called a nerve conduction test). And since we know how fast the wires should be and how many wires there should be, we can tell if there is something wrong with yours. We also put a little microphone into the muscles so we can listen to the talking going on between the nerves and the muscles (called an EMG). From listening in to this chat, we can learn if either the muscle or the nerve is having problems (because they complain!).

There are a lot of blood tests and urine tests (tests we do on your pee) that we can do to see how things are working; some of these are very special, and only a few places can do them. Finally, we may need to get a tiny piece of you to look at under the microscope, but this doesn't happen very often. Many of these tests are described again in the following sections.

Meet the Authors

The children in this book have been to a neurologist because either their brain has been sick, or they were born with a brain that didn't work like everybody else's. Some of the children don't have a problem with the brain but have a problem with their nerves or muscles. They want to share their stories with you so you can understand how they feel. If you got this book because you also have these problems, I hope that by reading these stories, you will learn that there are others out there who have gone through the same things that you are going through. And if you got this book because you know someone whose brain (or nerves or muscles) is different, you will see that these kids are really just like you. Finally, I hope your parents and teachers will read this book so they can understand better what it's like to be *you*.

I also want to say that these kids have taught their doctors much about the brain, about being sick, and about life itself. In fact, there is an eight-year-old boy who was taken to many doctors because he was "slow"–slow moving and slow thinking. When he saw his neurologist, she asked him, "Why do you think you are slow?" And he said, "Because that's the way God made me." This is an incredibly smart statement, and it came from someone that everybody thought was "dumb."

The best part of the book is that now, fourteen years later, these same children (now adults) want to tell you how they are doing (one person lives and works in Hawaii, and another in Germany!) and that their illnesses weren't the end of their lives but just a part of their lives.

THE DISORDERS

COMMON NERVOUS SYSTEM PROBLEMS

Epilepsy and Headaches

SEIZURES AND EPILEPSY

What Is a Seizure?

REMEMBER THAT THE brain uses electricity to talk to itself and the rest of the body. Sometimes that electrical system can short-circuit (almost like an electrical storm in the picture below); and when that happens, we call it a seizure.

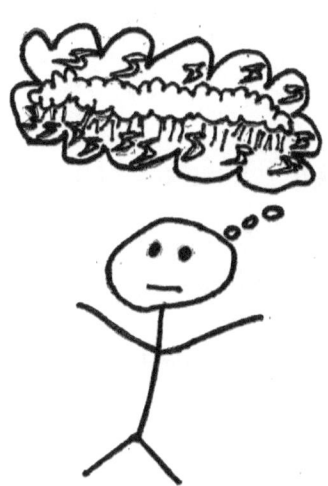

A seizure can last for a long time or be so short that nobody can tell when it happens. It can take up the whole brain or only involve a small part of the brain. It is not easy for the brain to talk to itself or the rest of the body during this electrical storm, which is why people can't think or talk well during a seizure. If the seizure is a big one, people fall to the ground, and their bodies shake, and they may drool and wet their pants. These are called generalized seizures. Another old term is grand mal seizures. If the seizure is a small one, they may only stare, and maybe just one part of their body may shake. People having these types of seizures will often do the same thing over and over again (just like a record that gets stuck!). Sometimes it is hard to tell that these people are having a seizure. These are called focal seizures.

What Causes Epilepsy?

People can have a seizure for a lot of reasons, including having a fever, not getting enough sleep, having an injury to the head, or taking the wrong medicine. Epilepsy means that a person has many seizures, and often we are not sure why. Many people have epilepsy because other people in the family have epilepsy (remember those things called "genes"). In other people, an infection of the brain can cause epilepsy. An injury to the head (remember the helmet!), a tumor, or a part of the brain that did not form quite right can all cause epilepsy. Sometimes there does not seem to be a reason at all!

How Does the Doctor Tell if a Kid Has Epilepsy?

A doctor can do many tests to see if a person has epilepsy. The most important is an EEG (electroencephalogram). An EEG measures your brain's electricity and looks for any tiny electrical storms. This is done by putting many wires on your head, and the electrical power of your brain sends a signal to the machine. By examining these signals, doctors can tell if you are having a seizure or if you have a brain that might have seizures. A CT scan (computerized axial tomography) is a special picture of your brain that looks for tumors. Sometimes another picture is taken, called an MRI (magnetic resonance imaging). This is a giant magnet, so the patients can't wear any metal when they have their picture taken (or they will stick to the machine!). You can tell which is which by what the machine looks like. The CT scan machine looks like a noisy giant doughnut, and the MRI is a noisy giant tunnel. There is a picture of an MRI in the **General Introduction** section. Sometimes the doctor might have to look to see if there is an infection around the brain that caused the seizure, and to do that, they have to take some of the fluid from around your brain. Most of the time, the doctors take the fluid from the back. Finally, blood tests can tell doctors if anything is wrong in other places besides the brain.

What Kinds of Seizures Are There?

There are a lot of different kinds of seizures. Some children have partial seizures. It starts in one part of the brain, and then it spreads. Depending on where the seizure starts, kids can have funny feelings that warn them they are about to have a seizure. One kid described that he felt scared when he had a "little seizure" and that he had a funny feeling that told him that he would have a seizure. But he takes his medicine and that helps. Another child stated that he fears his own fears. And for this child, the fears are worse than the seizures themselves.

Some children have absence seizures, which one kid described as having an antenna that breaks and then is fixed. For a few seconds, the brain is unable to do anything. Kids will stare blankly and may repeat things over again, like opening and closing a purse. This just lasts for a short time, and the kids won't realize that anything has happened. But they will have missed important information–like "go to the next problem" or "turn the page." So they will look confused when the world seems to have gone by without them. While each seizure lasts only for a few seconds, some kids can have over a hundred a day, so that can really add up! People with absence seizures can also have generalized tonic-clonic seizures (the kind where people fall down and shake all over).

How Do They Treat the Seizures and Epilepsy?

There are many good medicines that the doctor can give you that will help control the seizures. Most of the time, the medicine can make the seizures go away completely. Sometimes, you may still have a few but not nearly as many as without the medicine.

But the different medicines can have side effects. These are bad things that the medicines can do at the same time that they are doing the good things they are supposed to do. All medicines have side effects. Some medicines can make you sleepy or sad or behave badly. Some can make you want to eat more (and sometimes get fat). And some can make you hairy, while others can make you lose your hair. Many can affect the liver (which is an important organ that cleans your blood). That's why a doctor may need to check your blood while you are on some of these medicines. All of them can make you feel tired.

Don't worry; the doctor will talk to you about which medicine he or she feels is right for you. Sometimes the first one isn't the best, and we have to try another. But it is very important that you remember to take your medicine! The medicine cannot stop seizures if it stays in the bottle! Do you have to take medicine for the rest of your life? Maybe not. After we see that you haven't had seizures for a while, then we think it might be safe to try taking the medicine away. But this must be done slowly! *Never stop taking your medicine without your doctor's permission!* Bad things can happen, like you could have a very long seizure. So let your mother know if you spill the pills, for example.

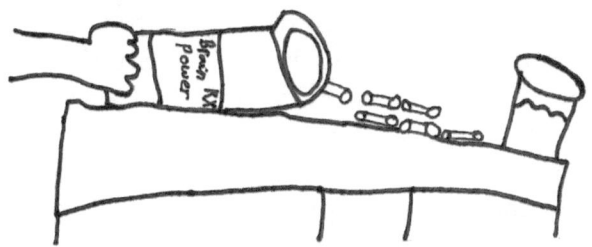

And you should let the doctor know how you feel. Some patients are anxious to get rid of their medicine; some want to keep taking it. Because you can't drive if you have seizures, a lot of patients want to stay on their medicine so they can get a driver's license when they get old enough.

What Do I Do if One of My Friends Has a Seizure?

Don't be afraid! Most of the time, the seizure will stop by itself. Although it might look scary, the person is not dying. Find an adult. Put a pillow under their head. Turn their face to the side. Do not put anything in their mouth! Do not hold them down, but take away anything near them that they might hurt themselves with.

What Can I Do if I Have Epilepsy?

Anything! Kids with epilepsy are just regular kids. They can do anything a regular kid can do. Did you know that famous people like Julius Caesar and Napoleon Bonaparte had seizures? Kids with seizures can be doctors and lawyers and teachers and parents. But most of all, they can be very good friends!

Voices of the Kids

Below are essays written by three children with epilepsy: Ashlyn, Geniece, and Ashley. It is also important to remember that the brothers and sisters of kids with epilepsy can also be confused and need to understand. Lana, who painted the picture used on the cover, talks about what the picture means and her need to understand why some people in her family have epilepsy and some do not.

Meet Ashlyn

In 2000 (Ashlyn was fourteen when she wrote her first essay). Ashlyn was nine when she started to behave in a strange way. She couldn't help it, but people just didn't understand why she couldn't control it. It was almost two years later that she finally had some answers. Ashlyn has partial seizures–or seizures that start in one part of the brain before spreading to the whole brain. These can be very hard to find and can make people act weird. Then, just as the seizures became better controlled, Ashlyn started to have dizzy spells, which turned out to be bad headaches called migraine headaches (migraines are described in the next section on headaches).

In 2014 Ashlyn has had a rough road but still looks to the future.

Complex Partial Seizures

In 2000

My name is Ashlyn. I am 14 years old. I have blue eyes, brown hair, and a wonderful, friendly personality.

I have epilepsy, migraines, dyslexia, and Attention Deficit Hyperactivity Disorder. I feel it is a lot that normal teenagers don't have to deal with. I do not like school much, however I like the friends I have at school.

Back when I was in 2nd grade, I starting screaming. It happened first when I was just waking up in the morning. Then it also started happening sometimes when I went to sleep at night. My mom did not know what it was. She thought I was doing it on purpose, but she brought me to my doctor. When he did not know what it was, he made me see a neurologist.

It feels weird. It feels as though you are in a dream and just cannot wake up. I scream and I cannot make myself stop. I can walk and move around, but it's like I am not really there.

When we went to the neurologist, I had a lot of tests. One was an EEG. This test is where they glued electrodes to my head. They didn't have to shave my hair. They just moved my hair as much as they could and glued it under it. I also had a MRI. This machine was like a rocket. I had to keep very still inside of it. All these tests came back fine. They sent me home and later I came back to the hospital for another EEG, but this time they videotaped me. I stayed for a long time, about a week. They still did not find anything. They put me on medicine because my doctor really thought I was having seizures, just none of the tests would show it. But I would still scream. One day while I was at school, I started screaming again. My mom picked me up and we went to the hospital in my town and they did another EEG. This time though I got to come home with the electrodes glued to my head. They were also connected to this little box. Every time I would eat, drink, sleep, or scream I had to press the blue button on the box. This time my doctor finally found out that I had seizures for sure.

They put me on some more medicine and I hardly have any seizures anymore. But sometimes I feel very tired.

The hardest thing about having seizures is frightening everyone when you have one. My little brother and sister really cries when I have one. They run to my mama and papa like I will hurt them. I guess when they get older, they will understand I will not.

Some things that worry me about having seizures are my ability to get rid of them, because I will not be able to drive unless I am seizure free for at least 6 months. Also, the possibility of not being able to have kids, because of the medicine I take.

However, the kids at school react in all different ways when I would have a seizure in class. Some would be worried, others scared, and others would ask questions. But the teachers were really nice and always seemed to handle things well. But I hated having them at school, because I'd get really tired and would have to check out. But I would usually feel better the next day or so.

I end this story with hope for other people with seizures, and also for them to know that life for people with seizures are only somewhat, very little, different then people without seizures.

Ashlyn

In 2014

I did finish high school, but was unable to graduate, because of secondary issues, memory problems. Therefore, making it impossible to pass the GEE 21, which is necessary to graduate.

Later when I was approximately 18 years old, the auras which were followed by seizures became more frequent, sometimes 3-4 times daily. Then, later in my twenties, the seizures were more severe, enough to compromise bladder and bowel control, which naturally became very upsetting to me, because they were not happening at home only. They were happening in public when shopping, eating at a restaurant, etc.

During these seizures, my grandmother would have to hold me up. I then began to limit my outings. My life became one of solitude, because I was afraid the seizures would happen in public. So, staying home was all that was comfortable to me.

My neurologist in Lafayette, LA at the time said that he could not help me anymore. He suggested I see a neurologist in New Orleans, LA at the LSU clinic. I was referred to [a doctor]. He evaluated me, and began treating me with medications, adjusting current, medications, and then he began trials on newer medications. All of his efforts still were unable to control my seizures, and make life better for me.

At that point he discussed brain surgery with me, and asked if I would consider it. It took me a couple of years to decide. I was also having to convince the important people in my life, because they feared the surgery would leave me in a vegetable state. They, however, did not understand just how miserable my life had become. I was ready to go anywhere, or do anything.

I agreed to an evaluation, and [the doctor] sent me for a consult with [another doctor]. She did a preliminary evaluation. Then, told me that she could make a decision only after an inpatient videotaping, where I stayed in the hospital and wore EEG electrodes for 4 days. I only had one seizure during the day, but had several during the night. It gave them information that was useful to be able to determine, if I would be a candidate for the surgery. I also had a MRI, functioning MRI, and a VEP, which also helped in the determination. The testing revealed that I had abnormal brain tissue patches throughout the left side of my brain, which was missed on every previous MRI. This showed the reason for my seizures, which gave me understanding, and acceptance of the situation I was now facing. The test had also revealed to the doctor that all of my functions, such as walking and talking, was not on the left side of my brain, like a normal person. My brain had stored the function of these on the right side of my brain, which made me an even better candidate for the surgery.

Consults were then scheduled with the two neurosurgeons, who would be performing the actual retraction.

I was admitted to [the] Hospital on July 28, 2014. On that day, they took me off all my seizure medications. They removed my skull on the left side, and put a grid of electrodes, which was attached to the left side of my brain. They refrigerated my skull that was removed for 5 days, while they collected data to use during surgery. The doctors were trying to find the correct origination point of my seizures in the abnormal tissue to retract. After collecting data for 5 days, on August 1, 2014, four doctors done surgery to complete the retraction. Although there are several patches of abnormal cells that still remain, they were able to remove the correct origination point and enough of the abnormal cells around it to reduce my seizures. Although I still remain on one anti-seizure medication, for the first time since I am 7 years old, I am seizure free!!!!!! I am going to be 28 years old on November 9th. I have not as of yet gotten my driver's license, however I am looking forward to that in February. Although [the surgeon] has made it clear that they were unable to remove all abnormal cells, and those could also develop into seizures, I am living my life today as a seizure free woman, looking forward to finally leading a normal life.

Meet Geniece

In 2000 (Geniece was eleven when she wrote her first essay). Geniece had her first seizure at age five. It was a very long one (called status epilepticus), and she was given phenobarbital. Phenobarbital is a very good medicine, but it sometimes can make kids behave in a weird way. This happened to Geniece, so she was switched to another good medicine. She is now almost twelve and is doing great. She had one seizure a couple of months ago because she forgot to take her medicine. She wants to be a pediatrician, so maybe someday, your kids will go to her!

In 2014 Geniece is a beautiful young woman. She graduated from Westgate High School in 2007. She went on to college at the University of Louisiana at Lafayette. She graduated from there with her BS in 2013. She currently lives in Lafayette, Louisiana. She is currently a case manager for the Lafayette Parish Office. She helps individuals who are incarcerated and have a drug or alcohol addiction transition back into society. She loves it and has found her true passion. Her ultimate goal is to get her LSW and is currently working on getting into graduate school now.

Geniece

Status Epilepticus, Primary Generalized Seizures

In 2000

Hi. My name is Geniece. I am a 12-year-old that has Epilepsy. The first time I had a seizure I was 4 years old, my mom had a garage sale at my aunt's house. My mom decided we should sleep at her house since the sale started so early in the morning. When I woke up the next morning I was shaking, drooling, and my eyes were crossed. When my sister DeLannie saw how I was acting, she called my mother. When my mom came into the room she said to call an ambulance. The ambulance took too long, so my mom, my nanny, and my aunts rushed me to the hospital. When I got to the hospital they ran all kinds of tests on me such as a catscan and an EEG. I had to stay in the hospital a few nights, so they could make sure I was O.K. I came home from the hospital and had to start taking some medication every day.

At first I did not like the medication, but I got used to it, it is really not that bad. Epilepsy is a scary word to the people that have it. The definition is very hard to explain, but you have seizures and I have mine when I am asleep. I don't get them very often but when I do it seems like I am having a nightmare and I am on a roller coaster. But when I take my medicine I don't have any seizures. Sometimes I forget, and I would like to thank my Daddy for reminding me to take my medicine. I would also like to thank my mom, sister, grandmothers, and my grandfather. It was really scary at first, but my doctor explains everything to me, and make sure I understand what is going on in my brain to cause me to have seizures. To everyone whom has epilepsy remember to take your medicine and your doctor will help you through this. You are not alone.

Geniece

In 2014

I am now a 25 year old that is living with Epilepsy. Whenever I tell people that I have Epilepsy, they ultimately throw up a red flag. Yes, I have Epilepsy, but it is not the end of the world. Every person who has Epilepsy is different. Some have mild seizures and others have severe seizures. Some have seizures every day and others have seizures rarely.

In my case, I only have seizures while I sleep. I have realized that the main cause of my Epilepsy is stress. Every time I would have an exciting event or a tragic event in my life, I would get a seizure. That caused a light bulb to go off in my head. Now I try my hardest to live a stress free life so that I can be seizure free. My last seizure was 4 years ago. So therefore, I know I am doing something right.

In my 21 years of having Epilepsy, people have said that I would not be able to do certain things, such as drive, hold a job, or go to school. These were just a couple of the many barriers that people were putting on my life. I was determined to prove these people wrong. I am now a college graduate who is working to get a master's in Social Work. I have a job that I absolutely love, helping individuals with drug and alcohol addictions. I have my supportive parents and family to thank for that.

It is up to you to learn about your own case of Epilepsy. And once you do that, you can manage your life much better. No matter how many times you are told that you can't, I am telling you that YOU CAN!!!!

Meet Ashley

In 2015 (Ashley was twelve when she wrote her first essay). Ashley is another girl with seizures. While she spends some time talking about the difficulties she has, she spends most of the time talking about the things she can do! And while her brain has "hiccups," it is special!

In 2015

Hi Everyone! My name is Ashley and I am 12 years old. I have had epilepsy for almost five years now. My first seizure was when I was 7 years old. It really scared me and my mom the first time it happened. I don't remember very much except having trouble talking and being very very tired. It was scary. Since then I've had lots of tests on my head and I have to take medicine every day. My doctor says my brain is different from other kids because of my "brain hiccups". I have to have someone watch me all the time in case something happens. I have trouble doing certain things and sometimes people don't understand me. School is very hard for me and it takes me awhile to learn things and sometimes I need things repeated to me because I forget. I get therapy at school to help me do better. I am tired a lot and usually sleep about ten hours a night. My parents check on me a lot as my seizures are more often at night time. I'm so glad for my mom and dad and my little sister, Alyson. Even though I struggle with activities I enjoy dancing the most. It takes me longer to remember the steps but I do my best when I perform on stage. I try to be as independent as possible and I even take the bus all by myself to school. The words in my head race sometimes and it's hard to concentrate, my doctor says it's because my brain is so "special". My mom is a nurse so I'm so glad she is so smart to take care of me. We carry special medicine if I have a seizure when we go places and my mom always keeps it in her purse. Other things I like to do is art and I love to color and paint. I want to be a teacher when I grow up. I have a few pets and enjoy playing with them.

Meet Lana

In 2015 (Lana was seven when she wrote this essay). Lana is the artist who provided the cover art called *Dog Not Knowing*, painted when she was six years old. She is the sibling of two family members with seizures. Below is her explanation of *Dog Not Knowing* in her own words. She explained to her mother that she was the dog and that she didn't know why her sister and she didn't have seizures but that her older two siblings did. She woke up one night to her sister having a seizure and then woke her dad to help. From that day forward, she felt that it was her responsibility to protect her sister. That is what led her to the art camp at the epilepsy foundation. She has always loved art, and her mother was hoping she would work through some of her feelings in the process of making art.

In 2015

I chose to paint this picture because I was confused that my brother and sister had seizures but my other sister and I didn't have seizures. I'm so happy that my sister isn't having a lot of seizures.

-Lana (aged seven years)

Lessons for Adults

A lot of children with epilepsy are more concerned about how others would see them than the fact that they had epilepsy. They commented on being worried that other kids would be scared of them or make fun of them. They were also afraid that people around them would not know what to do if they had a seizure. Kids have told me that their teachers have panicked and didn't know what to do. Therefore, it is not only sufficient to educate the patients with seizures and their families, we must also work harder at educating teachers, classmates, coaches, scout leaders, and other adults and children who are likely to interact with these kids. Even physicians need to be taught. One child suffered symptoms for months before anyone believed her. Even after discussion with her primary neurologist that there was an organic basis for her complaints, one consulted specialist still insisted that this was "all in her head." Classroom discussions, perhaps led by the children with epilepsy themselves, should be encouraged.

In addition, we need to foster a feeling of independence in these children, often difficult because of parental concerns (appropriate but sometimes stifling). As the child grows older, we discuss clearly the importance of allowing the child to have time away from parents to spend with friends. What works most often is a compromise: as long as the child wears a medic alert necklace, he or she may be allowed to indulge in age-appropriate activities.

Parents may also relax more if they are comfortable that their child's friends know how to manage in the event of an emergency. Geniece asked her doctor what to do if she should have a seizure. Apparently, Geniece's friend wanted to make sure that she knew how to take care of Geniece during a seizure. We must continue to emphasize that epilepsy is simply another chronic medical condition like asthma or diabetes. Only in this way can we reduce the stigma associated with this condition.

Finally, we have to remember that siblings are also often confused and want to understand better what is happening. Lana, who has a brother and a sister with seizures, talks about this confusion and expresses this in her art.

HEADACHES

Migraines, Tension Headaches, Chronic Daily Headaches

Why Do I Get Headaches?

THERE ARE MANY different kinds of headaches and many different reasons to have headaches. The most common headaches are migraines and tension headaches.

What Is a Migraine?

Migraines are very painful, usually pounding, and can make people sick to their stomachs (sometimes they throw up). Kids having migraines don't like being in bright light, and noise bothers them. Sleep is the one thing that can help, but some medicines can help too. We don't exactly know what happens to the brain to cause a migraine. We know that during a migraine, there are chemical changes in the brain, electrical changes, and we think maybe the blood vessels get too small to carry enough blood to the brain. Now, this isn't good for the brain, so it sends a signal back to the blood vessels and tells them to open up. Sometimes the blood vessels open up too big, and the blood rushes in too fast. This is what makes the head pound. It often affects the part of the brain that makes you vomit, which is why a lot of people with migraines get sick to their stomachs. So what kind of things can make you have a migraine? The most common thing is stress, like when you are worried about a test. Another common cause is certain foods like cheese and chocolate.

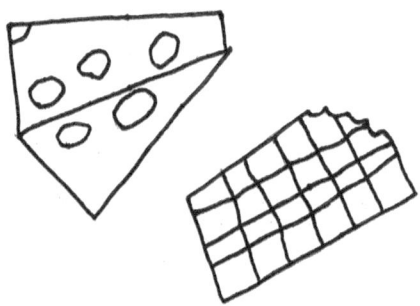

Sometimes exercise can do it. It is usually a little bit different for each person, and it is very important to try to figure out what makes it happen to you.

Who Gets Migraines?

A lot of people think only adults get migraines, but they are wrong. Do you know that they can happen in babies? So they can happen to any kid. But they are much more likely to happen to kids who have a mom or dad (or other family members) with migraines since they can be inherited (there are those genes again!). Very young children sometimes don't have any pain in the head at all but get dizzy or have stomachaches, and older kids can get confused instead. These are all considered migraines. Sometimes, little kids with stomachaches or dizzy spells have headaches when they get older. Someone with a migraine can also feel dizzy and "black out" and sometimes see funny things, like dots or lines, along with their migraines. There are some people who get the "numbies" and "tinglies" (like when your foot falls asleep), and very rarely, some people can't move one side of their body while they have a headache! Some people have a very funny way of seeing–things seem too big or too small. These are called changes in perception (the way we see things). Remember in the story of *Alice in Wonderland*, where Alice ate cake and drank tea and got really big and really small?

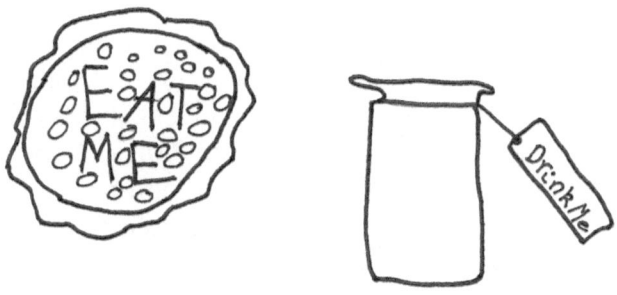

Well, that's because the author, Lewis Carroll, had migraines and had these changes in perception. So now in medicine, we call it the Alice in Wonderland syndrome. And don't worry. Most often, these problems go away when the headaches do.

What Are Tension Headaches?

Tension headaches are also known as muscle contraction headaches. These happen because there is a reflex that makes the muscles tighten when something hurts. This is so the muscles can act to protect an injured area. For example, if you fell and broke your leg, your muscles would tighten to protect the leg and hold the ends of the broken bone together. The problem is that it takes a lot of energy for the muscles to stay tight. The muscles can make the energy they need, but while they are making the energy, something called lactic acid builds up inside the muscles, and that can make the muscles hurt worse (which makes them tighten more!). So you can see how these headaches can be very hard to get rid of. Some people who have migraines have these headaches too. Sometimes it can be hard to tell the difference, but telling the difference is important. Medicine is often used to treat migraines, but muscle-stretching exercises can help the tension headaches.

The Ultimate Headache: Chronic Daily Headaches

When a person has a headache every day for a long period of time (one man I know had it for forty-five years!), it is called a chronic daily headache. These are the most difficult to treat because they can actually be a combination of three different headaches: migraines, tension headaches, and a headache called rebound headache. Rebound headaches are headaches that are caused by a lot of the stronger pain medicines. The medicine seems to work, and the headache goes away but comes back as soon as the medicine wears off. Taking more medicine only makes these headaches worse. So to get rid of chronic daily headaches, each of the three different headaches must be treated separately.

Very Rare Causes of Headaches

One of the most serious causes of headaches and the one that everybody is concerned about is a brain tumor. And while brain tumors are the second most common cancer in children (leukemia, a cancer of the blood, is first), they still don't happen very often. Infections of the brain can cause headaches, but a person with a brain infection will feel sick. Sometimes too much pressure builds up in the brain (usually because of too much fluid), and that can cause headaches. If you bleed into your head from an accident or because of a broken blood vessel, you can also get a headache as well as have problems with thinking and talking.

How Can the Doctor Tell What Causes Your Headaches?

As you can see, there are many different kinds of headaches, and your doctor needs to be able to tell what is causing your headaches and what type of headaches you have. Then they can figure out the best way to treat them. The doctor can take a picture of your head (either a CT scan or MRI) to look for a tumor or other physical causes like blood or too much fluid. He or she can check for too much pressure in your head by taking a look at the back of your eyeballs with a special light. Since your eyes are directly connected to your brain, if there is too much pressure in your brain, there may also be too much pressure in the nerve that goes to your eyes, and the doctor will be able to see that. Sometimes the doctor will have to measure the pressure, just like your dad measuring the pressure in the tires of your car. He or she will use a syringe to take out some of the fluid to relieve the pressure. This fluid can also be tested to make sure there is no infection. Removing some of the fluid very often makes the headaches a lot better.

How Are the Headaches Treated?

How the headaches are treated depends on what is causing them. If there is a brain tumor, the surgeon must remove it (see the section on brain tumors). If there is too much fluid and too much pressure, the doctor will need to remove the fluid and then give you a medicine to keep the brain from making too much. But in the rest of this section, I want to talk about how to treat the most common headaches: migraines, tension headaches, and chronic daily headaches.

How to Treat Migraines

The most important thing to understand is that there is only one person who can make migraine headaches better, and that is *you*! That is the most important thing–*you* have to take control! Don't worry though; doctors can teach you what to do.

Medicine is used a lot to treat migraines, and it comes in two forms. The first form is a medicine to prevent migraines. This is a medicine that you take every day to lower the number of migraines. I had one patient who was four when he developed bad migraines. I wanted to start the best medicine for him to prevent them, but it only came as a pill, and he didn't know how to swallow pills. Mom worked really hard to teach him how to swallow pills, but he just couldn't get the hang of it. Finally, Mom called to ask if there was a medicine that came in a liquid, and I said there was, but it could cause a patient to sleep more and eat more. Finally, the mom told the boy that if he couldn't learn how to swallow that pill, the doctor was going to have to start a medicine that would make him sleepy and fat. The next time he had a migraine, when it was over, he asked for his pills, and do you know what? He swallowed it right away! Since he started to take the pill every day, he didn't have another migraine. And he was so proud of himself that he had taken control himself. I bet that feeling of taking control was just as important to treating the migraines as the medicine itself. There are many different medicines that work to prevent migraines. Some affect the blood vessels, some are medicines for seizures, and some are medicines that are given to people when they are sad (antidepressants). Different medicines will work better for different people. So it is up to you and your doctor to decide which one is right for you.

The second kind of medicine is called an abortive medicine. This is the medicine you take if you already have a headache and need to stop it. The best ones are the simple medicines like ibuprofen and acetaminophen. But here is the secret: *you have to take the medicine within five minutes of the headache starting!* And since *you* are the only one who knows when the headache starts, *you* are the only one who can ask for your medicine on time! Many of these headaches start at school, but your mom or dad can fix it so you can take your medicine at school. You just have to let the teacher know. There are stronger medicines out there, but they can cause more problems. Sleep is one of the best ways to treat a migraine!

And finally, you need to keep going to school. Because every time you miss, you fall behind, and that can make you very worried. And the more worried you get, the more stress you feel, and the more stress you feel, the more headaches you will have. So *go*!

How to Treat Tension Headaches

Since these are caused by muscle contractions, the best way to treat them is to learn to relax the muscles. There are many ways to do this, but the best is something called biofeedback. In this therapy, they hook you up to a machine that tells you how tight your muscles are. The doctor then teaches you things you can do to relax those muscles, and you can tell which ones work for you, because the machine will tell you when you have gotten the muscles to relax. Pretty soon, you can do this without the machine. Other things that can help include massage therapy, stretching exercises, and finally, other relaxation techniques, like listening to the tapes of the rainfall or ocean waves (see, you always knew that music had to be good for something!).

When Things Get Really Bad

Since chronic daily headaches combine all three headaches: migraines, tension headaches, and rebound headaches, it is important to make sure to include the different treatments for all three—relaxation techniques and careful use of medicines—so that you can treat the migraines without causing the rebound headaches. Sometimes you might feel too weak to overcome these headaches. But you can reach down inside yourself and find all kinds of strength. It's important to know that *you can do it*! Some things that can help such as having quiet time or getting some exercise or doing other things you like to do to take your mind off your headache.

Myths

Sometimes, when headaches get very bad or start when kids are very young, people don't always understand. Many people, even doctors, believe that kids can't get migraines. Kids can be called crazy or mean or unhappy or be told that they are making it up. I saw one girl, at age seven, who was thought to be a bad person because she was so cranky and unhappy that she made everyone else around her cranky and unhappy. It turned out that she had been having migraines since she was an infant. She was started on some preventive migraine medicine, and she turned into a happy little girl. A lot of people think they are complaining so they can go home and don't have to do their work. But as you can see from this next group of kids, that isn't true at all.

Voices of the Kids

Below are essays written by three children with headaches: Steven, Laura, and Caine.

Meet Steven

In 2000 (Steven was sixteen when he wrote his first essay). Steven started having headaches at about twelve years of age. Then he began having dizzy spells along with his headaches, and they got so bad he could no longer go to school or do anything that he loved to do. He had seen a lot of doctors and tried a lot of different medicines, but nothing seemed to work. Pretty soon, some of the doctors were telling him that he was crazy. At age sixteen, Steven wrote about his headaches.

In 2014 Steven took a little more time to get back to me, as he is now living in Germany! Read the follow-up to his story and notice he is doing great!

In 2000

Incredible Pain

Imagine a red-hot needle being jabbed into your skull or being bashed in the head with a hammer. Have you ever experienced any pain similar to this? Well, I endured pain like this on a regular basis because of a terrible medical condition.

My nightmare began when, in the eighth grade, I developed a migraine condition. Migraines are severe headaches that occur when the blood vessels in the brain expand rapidly and then contract. This contracting of the blood vessels is what causes the intense pain. Migraines can be caused by any number of stimuli including stress, certain types of food, and blood hormone levels. Migraine conditions have also been linked to heredity. Needless to say, when I learned this I did some research and found out that I have a family history of migraines. The reason that I was unaware of this before is because migraine conditions frequently have gone undiagnosed in the past and even today.

Many people are under the impression that migraines are just severe headaches. For all migraine sufferers, I wish they were correct but sadly they are not. Along with the intense headache comes a plethora of other symptoms including nausea, blurred vision, hypersensitivity to light and sound, and vertigo. Having a migraine condition is like being a prisoner in your own body. The pain was so intense that I could not eat, sleep or even move. I would just lie there and do what

I could, which was not much, to bear the pain. The pain is so horrible that you want to die.

My search for medical treatment took longer and was more difficult than I could have ever imagined. First of all, my search for help began with my pediatrician whom I do not visit anymore because he accused me of faking my headaches just to get out of school. After my disagreement with my pediatrician, I began seeing a family internist. Fearing that he could not adequately treat my condition, he referred me to a neurologist in another town who unsuccessfully treated my condition and in turn referred me to another neurologist. By the time I received any successful treatment, almost a year had passed and I had seen four neurologists, four cardiologists, one endocrinologist, and countless emergency room physicians. Help finally came when my neurologist took away the fourteen pills a day that had been prescribed by the numerous doctors and giving me one "miracle pill."

I am proud to say that I have now been practically migraine free for three years. For this, I owe a debt of gratitude to my family for without them I never could have been able to overcome this major obstacle. Last but certainly not least, I would like to thank God for giving me the strength to overcome adversity. I hope that no one will ever have to go through what I did again. So to help make this dream a reality I plan on becoming a pediatric neurologist specializing in the treatment of migraines.

In 2014

As I look back on my "migraine year" several themes stood out. In particular, helplessness, skepticism and relief. Having visited so many doctors who were unable to help me as well as not being in control of my illness led to feelings of helplessness. Luckily my family supported me as we searched for treatment that would let me return to a normal life. The skepticism of several doctors, who insisted I was simply faking my illness, just added insult to injury. Again my family always supported me and were not swayed by this skepticism. Relief came in the form of a doctor who understood my condition and provided the only successful treatment I received. This treatment literally changed my life. After taking the medication for several years, I was able to stop the treatment and remain (almost) migraine free. Many years have passed since I stopped treatment and now only have migraine headaches two or three times a year. These rare occasions seem to be triggered by stress or disruptions in my sleep pattern. I am thankful for the unending support of my family, for finding an excellent doctor and for no longer being defined by this illness.

Steven

Meet Laura

In 2000 (Laura was eleven when she wrote her first essay). Laura was just 8½ years old and had had her headaches for over a year before she was referred to a neurologist. She has done a great job of learning how to control her headaches. She is now eleven and wants to share her experience with you.

In 2000

THOSE DREADFUL HEADACHES

Hi, my name is Laura. I am in the 5th grade and I am a straight A student. My mom's name is Claire. My dad's name is Paul. I have one brother and no sisters. Aaron is my brother's name.

It all started in 2nd grade. I was having headaches, very bad headaches. The headaches were mostly in the back of my head. Every time I had a headache at school, I would put my head down on my desk. It seems like most of my headaches started in the morning.

Sometimes they lasted about an hour or so, but other times they lasted much longer than that. They would sometimes make me feel dizzy, too. Sometimes the headaches got so bad that I cried at school. A few times I missed recess because of my headaches. I would stay inside and put my head down and close my eyes. A couple of times I fell asleep. When I had headaches during a test, I made lower grades. When the headaches got very bad, the school secretary would call my mom or dad to check me out of school.

Gymnastics is my favorite sport. But even though I loved it so much, there were times when I would miss it because of a headache. I can remember a few times being all dressed for gym class and on my way there, but I would fall asleep in the car and never make it to class. Mom would take me home and I would sleep for hours.

The first doctor I visited was my pediatrician. He couldn't find a reason for my frequent headaches. He suggested that I see a neurologist. Mom called and made the appointment.

On my first visit, my doctor took pictures of my head. I heard her say it was called a CAT scan. She took it because she wanted to make sure there was nothing in my head such as a tumor. She found nothing that would be as serious as a tumor. But she did find that I was having migraine headaches. She suggested that we start with only [ibuprofen] to see if it would help. My mom checked the [ibuprofen] into the school office. I had headaches almost every day and was going to the office for the [ibuprofen] often. One day the school nurse called my mom and told her I was taking [ibuprofen] way too much. On my next visit to my doctor she suggested a preventive medicine.

I started taking the [medicine] once every night. I didn't have to go to the office as much after that. My headaches started to slow down. As the headaches slowed down, they got less painful. I started making better grades on my tests and most of the time I could go to gym class without getting headaches.

During my third grade year, I visited the office less and less to get [ibuprofen]. Last year in fourth grade, I only went to the office twice the whole school year for [ibuprofen]. Now I am in the fifth grade and have only gotten [ibuprofen] once so far. I continue to take my [other medicine] once every night to help fight the headaches away. I am still making honor roll grades. I feel healthy and alive.

Meet Caine

In 2000 (Caine was seven years old when he wrote his first essay). When Caine was six years old, he was first being seen by the stomach doctors because of the vomiting that he was having. He complained of headaches too, but the doctors didn't pay much attention at first. He saw a stomach doctor who put a scope down his mouth so they could see what his insides looked like. Finally, they decided it wasn't a stomach problem and that maybe all his vomiting came from his headaches. That was when he came to see a neurologist. He is now seven and writes about his headaches.

In 2000

> Hi, my name is Caine Michael. I am seven years old. I like to sing, dance, draw and play sports.
>
> My headaches start with my eyes feeling funny, then I get nauseated, and my head feels like a rubber band is around it. Then it feels like my brain is getting knocked off and it hurts very bad and sometimes makes me cry. It feels like a big thundercloud came and whacked my head. Sometimes I throw up.

I had to go to the hospital to take a CAT scan and an M.R.I. The M.R.I. made very loud noises and it hurt my ears very bad.

Then we went to see a neurologist who said she had headaches too and they hurt.

When I get a headache I tell my Mom or Dad right away so they can give me some medicine. Then I go lie down in a dark room with a cold towel on my head.

I can't have chicken noodle soup anymore because it has an ingredient called MSG in it and this causes headaches.

My doctor said it is called a letdown headache.

If I want to eat the chicken noodle soup with MSG in it I have to take my medicine before I eat it.

Sincerely,

Caine

In 2014

I want you to know a few years after this the headaches stopped coming. I have since re-introduced foods containing MSG into my diet. The headaches haven't returned and I thank you for what you did back then.

PS: I still enjoy singing, dancing, and playing sports.

Lessons for Adults

Headaches, especially accompanied by vomiting, should always be taken seriously. Since school is the most stressful thing in most children's life, it is not unusual for them to get the headaches mainly on school days. Unfortunately, to a lot of people, this implies the kids are complaining of headaches only to avoid school. Also, we can see how young some of these children were when the headaches began. Migraines have been reported to occur in 5-20 percent of children and adolescents. Even though they were young, these children all were able to take control of their headaches once someone explained to them what to do. It is clear from these essays that as adults, we have a tendency to minimize both the amount of pain and the amount of stress these children are under.

Teachers, in particular, seem to have a problem with responding to their needs. One teacher told a parent that these headaches could not be migraines if they could be treated successfully by ibuprofen. Another informed a mother that it was not the teacher's responsibility to allow the child to get her medicine in the required amount of time, and if her headache got too bad, her doctor just needed to prescribe a stronger medicine. Unfortunately, many doctors do "help" by prescribing stronger medications with significant side effects and the potential for addiction. As the children explained, more and more medication is not the answer. The fact that these children can be so easily treated makes it that much more imperative that they are not ignored.

In addition, studies have shown that children as young as five worry about brain tumors. Doctors often don't want to mention it because they are afraid of scaring the children. Instead, the children are already scared, and we often are not doing a great job of reassuring them.

Finally, I have often had to emphasize that the headaches are the child's problem and not the family's. Mothers, in particular, can get over-involved. I remember one eight-year-old that had this problem. During the visit, I did talk to the mom about leaving him alone to sleep off the migraine in peace. When I saw them back, I asked the child how his mom was doing. They both laughed, and his mom said that with the very next headache, she started to do her "mom thing," and he told her, "Remember what Dr. Lee said?" He did admit that after that, she has done better.

NERVOUS SYSTEM PROBLEMS THAT CAN AFFECT BEHAVIOR

ADHD/ADD, Tics / Tourette's Syndrome, Autism

ADHD/ADD

"SIT DOWN!" "KEEP still!" "Stop talking!" "Pay attention!" Do you hear these all day long? Is it hard for you to concentrate on the math problems when that person in the front row is twirling her hair? Is it hard to sit still for hours while the teacher reads aloud from a book? Do you tell your best friend sitting next to you about the great game you got yesterday and then realize that in the middle of the math test was probably not a good time to talk about it? Are you someone that jumps off the roof–and then thinks about it on the way down? We call that impulsive. If so, then you probably have heard about those dreaded letters: *ADHD* (*a*ttention *d*eficit *h*yperactivity *d*isorder) is for kids who have trouble with attention and are too active (like a too fast car), or *ADD* (*a*ttention *d*eficit *d*isorder) is when a kid just has trouble with attention but is not running around all over the place.

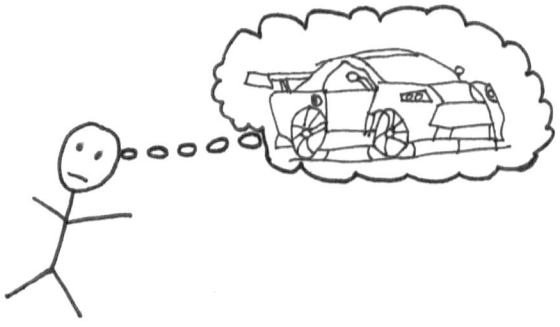

What Is Attention Anyway?

"Attention" is when you focus on one thing and ignore almost everything else. Another word for describing this is "concentrating." The brain does this by ignoring all signals that don't have anything to do with what the brain is concerned about at the moment. For example, while working on math problems at school, the brain will sift through all sorts of signals, like the heating fan starting up, the birds singing outside, and the person behind you coughing. The brain will decide that these are not important enough to drag you away from thinking about the math problems. But when the teacher says, "Time's up," the brain will note that this is an important piece of information (signal) and will shift your focus from the math problems to the teacher.

Some people find it easy to concentrate on one thing, while others find it very difficult. They would prefer to daydream than to listen to boring lectures. Also, their brains aren't good at screening out unimportant signals (or it makes a mistake and decides that some unimportant signals are important). Who are the kids that are more likely to have these problems? Well, boys, for sure. Boys' brains do work differently than girls', and when it comes to paying attention, girls' brains work a little better. Also, if one of your parents has a brain like this, then there is a good chance that you will too.

When Can It Be a Good Thing?

Some people believe that having ADHD-like behavior was very important to surviving in more dangerous times or places. It is better to be hyperaware of what is going on around you—like if you might be attacked by a wild animal as you approach the watering hole! (That's probably why boys' brains are better at being distracted—it was their job to remain alert to what was going on around them so they could protect people!) And people agree that there are certain jobs today where having these traits may still be important, like being a soldier, air traffic controller, emergency room physician, or salesperson.

So Why Can It Be a Problem Now?

Well, life has changed a lot in the past few hundred years. We no longer have to worry about wild animals eating us up in the grocery store. Also, everybody has to learn to read and write and do math if they are going to survive today. So everybody has to go to school and learn these things, and the only way we can teach everybody is to put them all in the same class all day long. So it is really hard for those brains that have trouble working with a lot of distractions around. That doesn't mean that your brain is stupid though!

How Can the Doctors Tell if You Have It?

There is no simple test for ADD or ADHD. The best way to see if you have it is to do an attention test. Some of these tests are fun because they are on the computer. Some are more old-fashioned and just require a pencil and paper. These tests are often given by special people called psychologists, but your school can give them too. These tests can be long, boring and seem to go on for days. But they can be very important because they give a lot of information about *you* and how your brain learns best, which can be very helpful. More often however, the doctor decides if you have ADHD or ADD by asking you, your mom, and your teacher if you have problems with attention (another way of saying you have trouble concentrating) or being too impulsive. (What is being impulsive? It's when someone jumps off a roof and then thinks about how this might not have been the best idea on the way down.) Sometimes a doctor will do an EEG to make sure you aren't "spacing out" because you are having seizures. Remember EEGs? These are the cool tests where they hook you up to a machine that can read the electricity that your brain makes. See the **General Introduction** section if you want to know more.

How Can Doctors Help?

There are some medicines that the doctor can give you that help your brain do a better job of screening the signals. The artist who has done all these great pictures inside the book calls her medicine Brain Power.

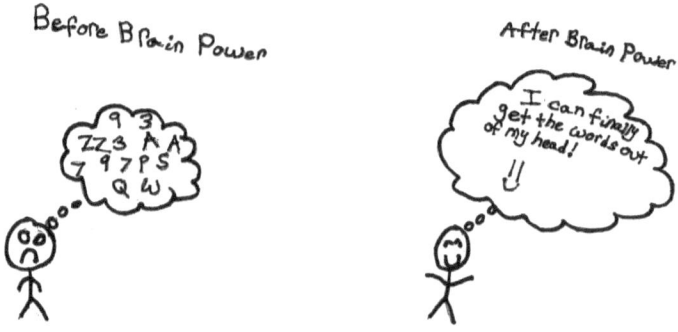

The medicine can help your brain decide which signals are important and whether it should bother you with them. That leads to better concentration. However, it is important to remember that these medicines can have side effects. Some can make you sad or make it hard to go to sleep at night. Some can cause tics (see the section on tics / Tourette's syndrome). Most of them can take away your appetite so you don't feel like eating.

How Can You Help?

You can help your brain become better at paying attention. How? It is just like how you teach your body to be a better soccer player–practice! Activities that are bad for teaching your brain how to pay attention include watching a lot of video games, using the TV remote control all the time, and Internet surfing. These things don't make your ADD or ADHD worse, but they don't help you to learn how to concentrate either. Activities that can help teach your brain include reading books, watching the history channel (minus the remote control), and conversation. Try it! Maybe if you get better at it, you won't have to take the medicine anymore.

Myths

People with ADHD are not stupid; nor are they bad kids. But you still need to learn to pay attention, and medicine is not the only (or even best) treatment.

Voices of the Kids

Below are essays written by two children with ADD/ADHD: Maddie and Spencer.

Meet Maddie

In 2014 (Maddie was eleven when she wrote this essay). Maddie had a difficult time reading and concentrating and did not like school. Her teachers were not very helpful or supportive in figuring out the best way to help Maddie learn. The school told Maddie's parents that she was dyslexic and that "nothing could be done." Dyslexia is when you have trouble reading because the letters get jumbled up. Her parents were not sure if she had ADHD because she wasn't a hyperactive child. The main symptom Maddie had was difficulty concentrating. Her parents were hesitant to start her on any medication, but school was getting worse for Maddie, so they felt like medication was their last and only hope. Maddie was started on a drug in May. The medication immediately helped her to concentrate and focus. Over the summer, she attended language therapy and a summer reading program through the local community college. As a result, Maddie jumped two full grade levels in her reading, gained a ton of confidence, and now enjoys school. Her parents wish they had started the medicine sooner!

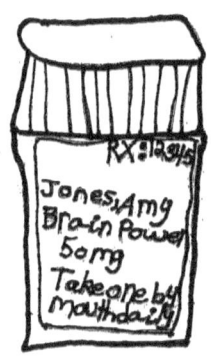

In 2015

My name is Maddie and I am 11 years old. I like the outdoors, playing video games, and playing with my friends. School was always hard for me. Words would scramble everywhere in my mind and I couldn't concentrate on any of my school work. Other kids in the classroom made so much noise that I couldn't focus to read or write. When I would read a book, the words would not make sense. I was very frustrated. When I did math problems, some of the numbers would jumble up. After I started [medicine], I could finally get the words out of my head! Reading and math are so much easier. I now love to read! I call my medicine Brain Power. Don't be afraid to try Brain Power. It has made a big difference for me!

Meet Spencer

In 2000 (Spencer was nine when he wrote his first essay). Spencer came to see a neurologist because of ADHD. He had been on one drug for a long time but didn't like taking it. His mother decided to try one of the natural herbs instead. But she did it very carefully and made sure Spencer's doctor knew what she was doing. Spencer was excited about getting off the medicine.

In 2014 Spencer was the furthest away of all the patients I contacted, enjoying life in Hawaii!

In 2000

> This is from Spencer. I would like to tell you how I got off of [the medicine]. My mother is trying something all natural. To see if I feel the same way. I know I feel better because my legs do not hurt any more. I just feel great. Because it is better to take something natural that is good for you. The best thing is that my doctor is on my side. Whatever I think is best for me. And I feel great taking something all natural.
>
> From Spencer

In 2014

Since then I am now a Sergeant in the Marine Corps and that's why I live in Kailua. It's really nice here I'm sure you remember. Been here over three years now, and just recently reenlisted for another four years. Trying to go recruiting next to move my career forward. My wife Heather and I are finally going visit this Christmas can't wait it's been about three years since. Honestly I forgot I was on [the medicine], but when I see your name it all came back. I think it's great what your book is trying to tell people with similar problems. When I stopped taking it I thought why I was ever taking that in the first place. I never had any problems after that.

Lessons for Adults

Of all the children that were asked to help with this book, the most resistance came from the kids with ADHD. While the other kids were excited about this project, to the child with ADHD, this request sounded like just more schoolwork. They had become so disenchanted with the whole educational process that even the possibility of becoming a published author held little appeal. It is also important to make sure that they have the time and opportunity to participate in activities that build up their self-esteem. While academics probably should be considered more important than sports, some leeway needs to be available. And while these kids can be very active, sometimes they are not the most skilled athletes. Also, the choice of which sport to play is important. Often, these kids are moving faster than their brains can keep up, so they can have a tendency to be clumsy. Therefore, it is vital to choose sports that allow for this.

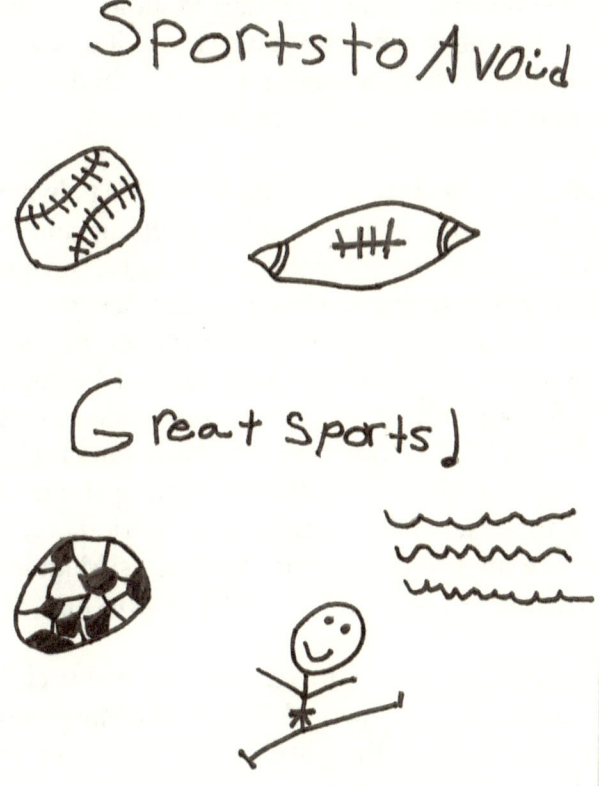

Sports that work well for these children include soccer (who cares if the child runs up and down the field four times while the ball has only crossed it once?), karate (there is an inherent sense of discipline established by an instructor who can break boards with his head), and swimming (it's hard to cut up with your face underwater). One sport to consider avoiding is baseball. These kids inevitably end up in outfield where very little happens. So the kids are busy watching the ants carry off a beetle when the fly ball finally does come their way. Don't ever ask a neurologist (especially a female one) about football.

What clearly separates a successful child with ADHD from a less successful one is their level of self-esteem. There was one parent who brought in tutors Monday through Friday to hammer in the basics. The recommendation of their neurologist was that they should concentrate on the basics Monday through Thursday but on Friday bring in someone to help the child grow his strengths (like art or music), not his weaknesses. All children need to have one area and time where they can be a star.

Stimulant medication is overused. We don't always appreciate the side effects; many have trouble sleeping and may require another medicine to bring them down at night. Most can suppress the appetite, which may affect body appearance (short and skinny), leading to a possible negative impact on self-esteem, especially during adolescence. Therefore, they should be used cautiously and with full knowledge of the potential side effects as well as benefits. But as Maddie points out, for the right child, they can be life changing. Usually, I recommend starting the medication but not telling the teacher. Then after a trial period, ask the teachers if they notice anything different. But just as Maddie says, often, the kids themselves will tell you that it is working.

Finally, it is important to realize that every child who has difficulty in class does not have ADHD/ADD. Many are hyperactive or distractible because the pace of the classroom is either too slow (rare) or too fast (very common). Stimulant medication will not make a child smarter. I remember seeing one kid who was diagnosed with ADHD and had been treated unsuccessfully with a stimulant. A neuropsychological examination revealed that he did not have ADHD. His behavior and school problems resulted from his unhappiness at living with his father instead of his mother. When these issues were sorted out, behavior and schoolwork improved without the need for medication. Therefore, it is vital that other diagnoses also be investigated before subjecting the child to long-term stimulant use.

AUTISM OR WHY DOES MY BROTHER ACT SO WEIRD?

What Is Autism?

WE SAY A person has autism when he or she has a lot of problems interacting with the people around him or her. Kids can have difficulty saying what they want to say, and some people with autism don't talk at all. They seem to want to play by themselves rather than with other kids, and sometimes they don't seem to care a lot about what other people think of them (although as you will find out, this isn't really true!). They may not be easy to teach to use the bathroom, and they have some weird behaviors. Sometimes they rock or spin, and if they get scared or nervous, they can scream and hit things or people (and it always seems to happen when you and your brother are at the mall and see your friends). A lot of kids with autism like to do the same thing over and over again. Some children with autism have a lot of trouble with learning. The first important fact about autism is that it is not a single disease. There are different types of autism with complicated names such as classic autism, pervasive developmental delay, and Asperger's syndrome. Although they may have different names, since they share the same characteristics, they are grouped together under the family name of autism spectrum disorders.

Some children are really bright, and they can do things that other people can't. They just have trouble understanding how to make friends. We call this Asperger's syndrome. But even some of the kids who have a lot of trouble with learning things, like spelling or reading, can do some things very well–like play music on the piano or remember a whole bunch of numbers. Sometimes it's hard to figure out how smart they are because they don't know how to behave around other people or understand when people say things to them. For example, what about the phrase "get out of here!"? If you say it with a mad voice, you're angry, and you want the other person to go away. If you say it with a smile, you may mean "you're joking!" Most people will be able to tell the difference because they can tell if you are angry or joking by looking at your face. However, to a person with autism, it will sound the same, and they won't be able to tell what you want them to do. It's important to remember that just because he doesn't act like he wants to be friends doesn't mean that he doesn't.

What Causes It?

Right now, we really don't know, although we do think that a big part may be due to heredity (again, with those pesky genes!), because it can occur in families. We do know that it happens in boys much more often than girls. Some people believe it might be because of eating certain foods or lack of certain vitamins or a certain infection or even because of the vaccinations. However, there has been no proof that any of these things can cause autism, and we do know for sure that it is not caused by vaccines. I believe that in people with autism, the brain formed differently from most other people's brains. Some of it didn't form as well, like the part that controls language, and some parts formed better, like the areas that help people remember things. Just like with any other group of people, kids with autism have their strengths and weaknesses too.

How Does the Doctor Decide if Somebody Has Autism?

The doctor will talk to the parents and also to the kid, if possible. The doctor can usually tell when the child learned to speak and how they behave if they have autism. Sometimes the doctor might do some tests if he or she thinks that there might be another problem causing the problem, but that will depend on what the doctor finds on the exam or while talking to the parents.

How Can We Treat It?

Right now, there is no cure for autism. Fortunately, a lot of kids with autism usually can be taught to talk and control their behavior. Sometimes medicine can help, especially if one of those behaviors is to hit people. It takes a lot of patience and love. Remember, even if he does act strange, he is still your brother!

Myths

Having autism is like being a square peg in a world filled with round holes.

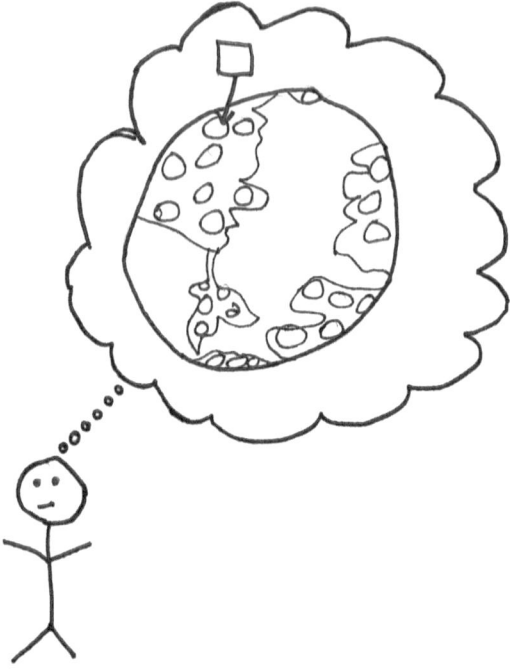

People with autism don't always fit in. So a lot of people think that kids with autism don't want to have friends, and because they act weird, other kids often pick on them. But you can help make it better. How? Listen. Sometimes kids with autism have unusual habits. One patient with Asperger's advises that if you don't understand what someone is doing or why, just ask. But be patient because sometimes, it takes a while for kids with autism to get their thoughts together. And sometimes they can get stuck on one idea. I had one patient that was told he had to wear a helmet when he rides his bicycle, and he insisted for his mother to stop that night on the way home to get one. And the next time he saw me, he proudly showed me a picture of him on a bike, wearing his helmet. I must admit, I wish that more of my kids had followed those directions so carefully! Try not to use confusing language, which can mean many different things. Kids with autism can like to focus on certain things and then learn everything they can about that one topic. I had one patient who loved *Star Wars* and could even draw all the engineering plans of the Death Star. So they can really help out with projects. Invite them to be friends. I had one patient who was sad that he didn't have any friends. He admitted that it wasn't that he didn't want to make friends but that he just didn't understand how. Don't tease them or pick on them because they are different. Instead, ask them why they are acting that way, and you will learn a lot. And maybe it's about time that we make sure that some of those holes are square.

Voices of the Kids

Below are essays written by four children with autism: Christopher, Ryan, Tyler, and Chance.

Meet Christopher

In 2000 (Christopher was fifteen when he wrote his first essay). Christopher is on a medication to help him focus and is doing great in school. He is looking forward to getting his driver's license. He sometimes gets anxious and is on another medicine to help him with that. As you can tell, he loves high school.

In 2000

Hi, my name is Chris. I am 15 years old and I have Autism. I have two sisters and one brother. I live with my mother and father and my sisters. I didn't begin talking until I was nine years old. I started school when I was three years old. It was a kindergarten school. I stayed there for three years. Then I went to an elementary school for five years. That's where I began to really talk. It's also where I made principle's list and honor roll. I also competed in Special Olympics, winning many ribbons. First, Second and Third places in running and throwing the ball the farthest. Then when I was 11, I went to a middle school. There I made good grades and met many people.

We would go to the bowling alley and in my last year there I won 3rd place. Now, I am in my first year of high school. I meet and talk with a lot of students and the coaches are my buddies. This year our class was in a bowling tournament and I scored a 180 and won first place. This year my brother let me drive his car in my yard with his help. I received a letter from the National Honor Roll United States Achievement Academy stating that I have been nominated as a member. I will be in the United States Achievement Academy National Awards Yearbook. I also love to play video games. I play one game until I beat it. Sometimes it takes me a few days to beat it. I also listen to rock music and my favorite band is Creed.

I think that I have come a long way from when I was a baby and couldn't talk. I have plans for my future. I want to get my driver's license next year when I turn 16. I also want to graduate from high school and attend college.

Meet Ryan

In 2000 (Ryan was ten when he wrote his first essay). Ryan was referred to a neurologist at age ten because the school wasn't sure if he had a learning problem or trouble with his nerves. He couldn't keep up in his private school, so he was transferred to a public school. It was the public school teachers that realized why he had a problem fitting in. He had a mild form of autism. He writes an essay here to tell you what he likes about his new school.

In 2014 When contacted, Ryan did not want to write a follow-up essay. But his mother writes that he is twenty-three years old and doing well. He has graduated from high school. He did not want to go to college because high school was difficult. Although on graduation night (2010), he was awarded Mr. Ville Platte High. The award is given to the student who works the hardest. Ryan has an interest in watching the news (*CNN*).

In 2000

What I like about School

I like my new school because I like to play with something on the playground we call the snake. When I sit on it, it moves side to side like a snake. I also like my school because I have the best teachers in the Universe. She helps me with my class work, and watches over me. When she is not there another teacher watches over me. I get to stay in her classroom for the day. Since my teacher helps me with my class work I don't have to study and do homework as much when I went to my old school.

Ryan

Meet Tyler

In 2000 (Tyler was seven when he and his mother worked on his first essay together). Tyler is seven and does have difficulties with talking to people. He is doing well on a medicine that helps his behavior and is being homeschooled. The homeschool environment is working so well for him that the medicine is being tapered. The first time his doctor met him, he liked to meow like a cat. He's not really talkative, so his mother interviewed him over several days for this book and recorded it for us.

In 2014 Tyler has come such a long way and is doing very well. His parents continued to homeschool him through high school, and he graduated in May 2013. He has had four jobs but has not yet found the right one. His dream job is to work on a creative writing team for monster/superhero movies.

In 2000

Child's Name: Tyler *DOB:* November 16, 1994
Age: 7 years old *Grade:* 1st Grade
School: Home Schooling *Teacher:* Mother

Date: Tuesday, December 4, 2001

Mother: Tyler talk into the microphone, ok. What's your name?
Tyler: What's your name.
Mother: No, Tyler. What's your name?
Tyler: What's your name.

Mother: No, Tyler. What's your name?
Tyler: What's my name.
Mother: Tyler, tell me what your name is?
Tyler: Tyler
Mother: Can you spell your name so she gets it right?
Tyler: T-Y-L-E-R
Mother: What's your last name?
Tyler: Tyler
Mother: Your last name is what?
Tyler: Tyler
Mother: When's your birthday?
Tyler: November 16th
Mother: 1994
Tyler: 1994

Mother: How old are you Tyler?
Tyler: 7
Mother: 7 years old
Mother: What grade are you in?
Tyler: November 16th
Mother: No, what grade are you in?
Tyler: November 2nd
Mother: No, you are in the 1st grade.
Tyler: 1st grade.
Mother: Yes, 1st grade
Tyler: Yes, 1st grade
Mother: Where do you go to school?
Tyler: …at… at. I don't know
Mother: You go to school at home?
Tyler: Yes.
Mother: Home school
Tyler: Home schooling
Mother: Who's your teacher?
Tyler: Mommy
Mother: Yes.
Mother: Then you go to Breaux Bridge Primary?
Tyler: Yes, Breaux Bridge Primary.
Mother: What do you do at Breaubridge Primary?
Tyler: Drive.
Mother: What do you do when you go to Breaux Bridge Primary?
Tyler: Uuh.
Mother: Whom do you go to see at Breaux Bridge Primary?
Tyler: People.

Mother:	What's her name?
Tyler:	Uuh.
Mother:	Who is your teacher at Breaux Bridge Primary?
Tyler:	Ms. [???]
Mother:	No, Ms. Chris.
Tyler:	Ms. Chris.
Mother:	Ms. Chris is your teacher. What does she teach you?
Tyler:	Uuh.
Mother:	She teaches you speech.
Tyler:	She teaches me speech.
Mother:	Speech Therapy.
Tyler:	Speech Therapy.
Mother:	Yes! That's a hard word to say.
Tyler:	Speech Therapy
Mother:	So, what do you like to do, Tyler?
Tyler:	I like to . . . watch movies and work in my lab.
Mother:	Work in your lab?
Tyler:	Yes.
Mother:	What is your favorite show?
Tyler:	Batman and Cubix for Everyone and some . . .
Mother:	Do you like to play outside?
Tyler:	Uuh, my Pokémon movies
Mother:	You like Pokémon movies?
Tyler:	Yes, Pokémon Movie 3. Yes, Pokémon Movie 3 and . . .
Mother:	All the robot kind of things
Tyler:	All the robot kind of things and like Power Ranger and everyone.

Mother: And, what else do you like to do besides watch movies, play with your Power Rangers and robots?

Tyler: And . . .

Mother: Do you go outside?

Tyler: And, I go outside.

Mother: What do you do when you go outside?

Tyler: Play!

Mother: With whom? Who do you play with when you go outside?

Tyler: My partners named Steven and Alex.

Mother: You like Steven and Alex. They're your partners.

Tyler: Yes.

Mother: But, when Steven and Alex are not there; whom do you play with?

Tyler: Mary and Rachel.

Mother: Your sisters, Yes . . . who else? Do you have any cats?

Tyler: I have a kitty cat.

Mother: How many kitty cats do you have?

Tyler: Two.

Mother: What are their names?

Tyler: Shadow and Moe.

Mother: Shadow and Moe.

Tyler: Yes.

Mother: Are they boy cats or girl cats?

Tyler: Boy cats.

Mother: Boy cats.

Tyler: Yes.

Mother: What else do you like to do?

Tyler: Work.

Mother: What kind of work you like to do?

Tyler: Batman, I am Batman.

Mother: You like the story?

Tyler: I am Batman and I was just saving the world.

Mother: You were saving the world?

Tyler: Yes and I jump and fly up in my Batman holder. I fly and bump somebody and I do some tricky jumps and I kick, do my arms like that and kick on the back, and now a spike hit.

Mother: You did a spike hit.

Tyler: Yes.

Mother: Are you happy?

Tyler: mmm!

Mother: You have to say "Yes" or "No". She can't see you shaking your head.

Tyler: Yes, yes.

Mother: What makes you happy?

Tyler: Watching "Spy Kids" at the movies. Yes, at the movies again and I have a belt with a machine on it and I was working and I was working. We have enough.

Mother: You've had enough? You have had enough working.

Tyler: Yes.

Mother: You don't like working for a very long time do you? Just a little short work and then you do something else.

Tyler: I was going to fix my machine and I have some purple beans that I cleaned off so they can be shiny again.

Mother: So they can be what?

Tyler: So they can be shiny and bright.

Mother: You were cleaning them with water?

Tyler: Yes.

Mother: Do you get mad sometimes.

Tyler: No.
Mother: Really, you never get mad?
Tyler: NO!
Mother: You never get mad when your sisters get you frustrated?
Tyler: No!
Mother: You don't get mad at them?
Tyler: NO!
Mother: So, you are happy all the time.
Tyler: No!
Mother: You are happy. You're very happy.
Tyler: Yes!
Mother: What makes you happy?
Tyler: We have had enough for now.
Mother: You have had enough for now?
Tyler: Yes.

Date: December 5, 2001

Mother: Today is December 5, 2001. This is Tyler again and we're not happy today. What is wrong Tyler?
Tyler: I am trying to go to bed.
Mother: Why do you want to go to bed?
Tyler: Because I am so tired and sick.
Mother: You're tired and sick?
Tyler: Yes.
Mother: What hurts?
Tyler: My head.
Mother: You have a headache?

Tyler: I want to go over here.
Mother: Why do you have a headache?
Tyler: Because, I have to go to bed.
Mother: Ok. We were fine until told that we could not watch TV. We have a headache now. We'll try again later.

Date: December 12, 2001

Mother: Hi, Tyler.
Tyler: Hi.
Mother: Do you get mad sometimes?
Tyler: No!
Mother: Sure you do, sometimes. Remember this morning you were mad. Do you remember why you were mad this morning.
Tyler: Yes.
Mother: Why were you mad?
Tyler: Because I wanted to go to bed.
Mother: No, you didn't want to go to bed. When we were in the car driving. Remember?
Tyler: Yes.
Mother: Why were you mad?
Tyler: Because I was had a headache.
Mother: Do you get many headaches?
Tyler: Yes.
Mother: Yes. What makes you happy? What do you like to do?
Tyler: Play and pet the kitty cat.
Mother: That's all you like to do – play and pet the kitty cat?
Tyler: Yes.
Mother: Where are you going tonight?

Tyler:	Martial arts.
Mother:	Martial arts class. Who is your teacher?
Tyler:	Master Keith.
Mother:	Master Keith, yes. Do you like martial arts?
Tyler:	Yes!
Mother:	Why do you like martial arts? What do you like about it?
Tyler:	I like doing kicks and . . .
Mother:	Do you like being with all the other children?
Tyler:	Yes.
Mother:	What's your favorite thing to do?
Tyler:	Play toys and Max Steel.
Mother:	Do you like going to school?
Tyler:	Yes.
Mother:	What do you like best to do at school? When you are at school, what do you like to do best?
Tyler:	I don't know.
Mother:	What do you not like to do at school?
Tyler:	I don't know.
Mother:	What's your favorite thing to do at school?
Tyler:	I don't know.
Mother:	Do you like to color?
Tyler:	Yes.
Mother:	Do you like to write your name?
Tyler:	Yes.
Mother:	Do you like to read books?
Tyler:	Yes.
Mother:	What kind of books do you like to read?
Tyler:	Power Rangers.

Mother: What other kinds of books do you like to read?

Tyler: I don't know.

Mother: Do you like to do math?

Tyler: Yes.

Mother: Do you like to do science?

Tyler: Yes.

Mother: What is science?

Tyler: I don't know.

Mother: Are you just saying what you think I want you to say.

Tyler: Yes.

Mother: But, that is not what I want. I want you to tell me about Tyler. What does Tyler like to do and what do you not like to do?

Tyler: I don't know. I don't know the first words.

Mother: The first word of what?

Tyler: Of being Tyler.

Mother: Of what Tyler likes?

Tyler: I just don't want to.

Mother: Ok, you don't have to get upset. It's ok. It's alright. You don't want to do this anymore?

Tyler: No!

Mother: Ok, tell Dr. Lee Good-bye.

Tyler: Good-bye.

In 2014

Information on Aspies, from an Aspie

By Tyler   11-10-14

1 Communicating - As a child, before I started speaking, my thoughts were so vivid that I thought I WAS speaking, but no one understood me. Then, at around the age of 4, I spoke in my grandmother's driveway and my family actually responded! In that moment, I remember raising my arms and saying "THEY UNDERSTAND ME!!!" So whenever you're trying to talk to your Asperger child and he/she doesn't respond, know that your child isn't trying to ignore you or doesn't want to talk to you, he/she just doesn't know how.

#2 Obsession has been my weakness, I grow too attached to things and it causes problems in the long run. If you can somehow teach your Asperger child to not become obsessive at an early age, then it will make life easier for both the child AND the parent.

#3 Education- I did 3 years of preschool plus kindergarten in the public school system, and 6th grade and 10th grade in a private school setting. The rest of the time I was homeschooled. I always found that homeschooling was the best option for me. As an Aspie, I required more hands-on, one-on-one instruction than was possible in a typical school setting. I had a hard time keeping up with the rest of the class and therefore was left behind, leaving me stressed and agitated. By mid-year I would give up on even trying to catch up because I saw no hope of it ever happening. However, when I was home-schooled, I had all the time I needed to keep up and my mom could modify my lessons to suit my needs. Most times tests were given orally, breaks were frequent, we took lots of field trips, and we watched lots of educational videos which I found more helpful than reading a textbook. This made for a more relaxed and adaptable learning experience. We also incorporated outside help with speech and occupational therapy and tutoring.

Meet Chance

In 2000 (Chance was seven when he wrote his first essay). Chance is seven and has a special form of autism called hyperlexia. This means he is very good with words and learned to read very early. He does have some problems with behavior, but he was started on medicine to help with that. When he was told by his neurologist that he had to wear a helmet when he rode his bicycle, he insisted that they stop on the way home to get one. The next time he came, he brought a picture of himself on his bike, wearing his helmet! His mother helped him put his thoughts and ideas into this essay.

In 2015 Chance took his time on his second essay as he looked back on the first, which he wrote so long ago. His follow-up essay is beautifully written and demonstrates a real talent for using words to convey important ideas. I feel very lucky to have the opportunity to share his thoughts and understanding with you.

In 2000

My name is Chance, I am seven years old and I have autism. I do not understand what this is, but I do know that it makes me different from others. I like playing with trains, riding bikes and playing video games. My favorite game is Pokémon because I really like the way the characters evolve into other forms. I think I am very good at my game boy color. I have a love for books and learned how to read since the age of two. I want to be a meteorologist when I grow up and have read many books on this subject. My mom always tells me that just because I have autism doesn't mean I can't be anything I want to be when I grow up.

Because I am different I don't have many friends. It's not that I don't want to make friends, but I don't understand how to make friends. Everyone should have a friend, just because I have a different way of doing things doesn't mean that I can't be a good friend. I don't like many types of foods, they feel weird on my tongue and taste yucky. My favorites are plain rice, sliced bread, cereal (no milk) and of course a plain cheeseburger from McDonald's. In the first grade I was in the school play and was chosen to sing the music solo, I liked that a lot.

I am now in second grade. I am in a regular classroom with everyone else so I don't feel so different there. I really love school and think I am smart. I make the honor roll and study hard. I was chosen to be in the school spelling bee.

Riding bikes is my favorite past time. Dr. Lee tells me you should always wear your helmet when riding a bike, so I do. I have a lot of pets like my 2 fish, one dog and seven cats that I love to spend time with. We are four people in my family my dad, mom, older sister and myself. I love my family, I know my family loves me and they do not treat me any different because I have autism. Autism is not like other disabilities. You cannot tell I have this just by looking at me. I am different and that's ok because remember God made each and every one of us in his likeness even though we may be different to the world.

In 2015

I had looked at the essay that Dr. Lee sent me before I wrote this follow-up essay, and I was amazed at how much had changed in roughly fourteen years. After all, life is full of changes. However, that does not mean that everything has changed- at least, not fully or more completely than not- but life does, indeed, have its changes. One can say that at least one of the purposes of writing this follow-up essay was to respond to the one that I had written when I was seven. I have certainly come a long way since then.

Autism makes me different mainly in the way that I communicate and process, and I did come to realize that, at least more and more, sometime as I matured. However, I do not believe that anyone- other than God- can ever fully understand autism, myself included. Autism is a part of me; I live with it, I accept it, and I do not fully understand it, but it does not have to define me. Rather, I let the fact that I am a perfect child in the eyes of God define me. Continuing on the subject of activities, hobbies, and whatnot, unless you count video games- which I have liked playing for at least most of my life, at least up to the point of when I completed this essay, and likely do still like playing-involving them or something along those lines or if I do so with a friend, with a relative, or whatnot for whatever reason, I do not play with trains or ride bikes anymore. I also do not like Pokémon anymore. As for reading, although I do not have nearly as much time as I used to for reading, I still like to do so. Although I no longer want to be a meteorologist, as I did when I was seven, I have always had- and likely still do have-an interest in weather- and natural disaster-related things. Finally, in response to the last statement in the first paragraph of the essay that I wrote when I was seven, it is true that just because one has autsim does not mean- at least when it comes to one's calling, I believe, anyway- that he or she cannot be anything that he or she wants to be when he or she grows up. When it comes to accomplishing things, autism is not necessarily an impenetrable wall, but rather, an obstacle that has to be overcome. When autism is indeed an obstacle, it can indeed be overcome.

Continuing in a similar vein, just because one is different does not mean that one cannot have many friends. Although I am still working on making friends, talking to people, strengthening relationships, and whatnot- all of these require continuous work, of course- I certainly have more friends than when I was seven. Friendship can be difficult to understand, at least at times, but I have picked up more understanding about it. I believe that everyone should have several friends. It does not matter if you do different things or do things differently when it comes to being a good friend; anyone can do it. I also believe that you do, however, have to choose your frinds wisely, especially when it comes to closer and closer friends. When it comes to food, I have certainly expanded my horizon; I now like many types of food, my favorites at the time of writing this essay being potato salad-without relish- jambalaya, fried butterfly shrimp, and perhaps others that I have left out. I also like some fruits such as bananas, blueberries, and, perhaps my favorite kind of fruit, raspberries, although my horizon certainly is not limited to the things that I have listed, although I do still like plain rice, sliced bread, cereal without milk-although when I eat it, I eat it with milk at least most of the time now- and plain cheeseburgers from McDonald's. As for the school play in the first grade, I honestly do not remember singing a solo, although I do remember, among other things, that it was a Christmas-related play and that I was one of the three kings bringing gifts to Jesus.

I began writing this essay when I was a junior at the University of Louisiana at Lafayette, and I completed it somewhat shortly after becoming a senior. A times, at least, I have felt that I was at least somewhat busy to the point of not working on the essay, at least, very often to at least some degree and- or alternatively, or- quickly to at least some degree. I have always been in regular classrooms, but notably, I took special keyboarding and handwriting-and whatnot, perhaps, which I have mentioned because I do not quite remember- sessions in elementary school and study skills classes throughout middle school and high school, and additionally- at least, again, at the time of writing this- I was enrolled in the Office of Disability Services and the Student Support Services programs at UL Lafayette. I believe that they have helped me significantly in my education. Like when I was seven and whatnot, in the regular classrooms, I have not felt so different, and additionally- again, like when I was seven and whatnot- I have liked school. I believe God has blessed me with wisdom and intelligence. Too, I believe, at least some degree of notability, I have achieved a 4.0 GPA in high school, and additionally- again, at least at the time of writing this- I have kept a 4.0 GPA at UL Lafayette. Other than once in the fifth grade, I have made the honor roll- and, I believe, the principal's list at times- throughout elementary school and middle school. As for the spelling bee, I was a participant in a spelling bee when I was in first grade; I believe I made it to the top three, but I lost when I misspelled the word "straight." "S-t-r-a-i-t," I believe, was the way that I spelled it; my late grandmother on my mom's side of the family got me a trophy, though. In one's life, there are ups and downs as well as victories and defeats, and I believe that most if not all people experience each or a combination of these at least once in life.

I have not ridden a bike in years, although I may ride again in the future. However, for one to wear a helmet when riding a bike is, I believe, good advice! As for pets, at least at the time of completing this, I had about, at least five guppies-fancy guppies, I believe- a small catfish- a cory, or perhaps Cory, catfish, I believe, but at least at the time of writing this essay, I did not remember if it is called a striped cory catfish, a spotted cory catfish, or whatnot-an aquatic tiger nerite snail, and a snapping turtle as pets. I like my pets. I am still in a family of four, but at the time of writing this, I have not lived with my sister for years, though I have still seen her at times. I still love my family, and I always will. My family still loves me, and I do not believe that there are very many, if any, differences in how I am treated due at least in part to me having autism. In response to the third- and second-to-last statements in the essay that I wrote when I was seven, I believe that autism is not like, at least, many other disabilities and that it is at least somewhat difficult to tell that I have autism by looking at me. In response to the final statement of the essay that I wrote when I was seven, I still believe that it is okay to be different. I believe that it is okay for me as well as anyone and-or alternatively, or everyone else to be different, though. I still believe that God, despite us being different to the world- I do not quite remember if, in that last statement in the essay that I wrote when I was seven, I meant "us" and "the world" either in the context of disabilities or in the context of what might call religious beliefs, but whatever it may have been, in the writing of this essay, I intended to make this statement in the context of my beliefs-made all of us in His likeness.

I wanted to conclude this follow-up essay with some additional information. For the work that I will have done during the course of my life, I will use the pen name- and, or alternatively, or, the nickname- C.K. Bourgeois. At least at the time of writing this essay, I was a Moving Image Arts major-that is, I primarily studies movie-making- and an English minor at UL Lafayette. I was living in Lafayette- or, perhaps, Scott, perhaps depending on how one views it- in Louisiana. My favorite band was- and likely still is- Fireflight, and my favorite video game was- and, again, likely still is- Kirby Super Star Ultra. Besides the Bible, my favorite book, or book series- in the case of my favorite book or book series other than the Bible, I won the entire series compiled into one book- is perhaps- and, perhaps, likely still is- The Chronicles of Narnia by C.S. Lewis. I have worked at least two jobs; one was as an usher at one of the two Grand Theater- or, perhaps, Theatre- locations in Lafayette and the other was as an audio and, primarily, video editor in TFC Media at The Family Church in Lafayette. Finally, God has called me to be a director and a writer, and I intend, during the course *of my life, to have done what I have been called to do.*

Lessons for Adults

It is easy to assume that because autistic children do not appear to pay attention to the people around them, they aren't interested in social interactions. While these kids do want to build relationships, in reality, it is the methods by which personal relationships are formed that can be incomprehensible to children with autism. In some respects, these children are like foreigners being dropped into an alien culture where they don't speak the language well and have no concept of the rules of the society.

One physician, who is an expert on autism as well as the mother of an autistic boy, offers guidance in dealing with these children. She suggests that the technique for making friends be broken down into a step-by-step process that provides a mechansim whereby the child may learn a small range of acceptable behaviors and when to use them. While this may limit flexibility, it will help prevent inappropriate responses in social situations. Accomplishments must be linked to tangible rewards since there is little motivation to complete a task to please others. It is very difficult to extinguish an inappropriate behavior, especially when the child finds it completely logical. Therefore, gentle attempts to substitute a more socially appropriate behavior, which still fufills the child's needs, should be encouraged.

As is often the case, the best advice comes from the kids themselves. Be patient, inquire as to the reason for unusual behavior, but most importantly, provide these children with every opportunity to fly.

NERVOUS SYSTEM PROBLEMS THAT AFFECT STRENGTH

Weakness (Myopathies, Neuropathies), Cerebral Palsy

WEAKNESS THAT EVEN A WHOLE LOT OF SPINACH WON'T HELP

Myopathies, Neuropathies

What Determines Strength?

SOME PEOPLE ARE just stronger than others. So what determines strength? Well, it's a combination of the size of the muscles (boys' muscles are usually bigger than girls'), the nerves that carry the information to tell the muscles to move, and finally, the brain that controls the whole thing. Weakness due to brain problems is talked about in the next section on cerebral palsy. Here we will talk about being weak because there is something wrong with the nerves or muscles.

What Happens When the Nerves Don't Work Right?

Nerves are the wires that carry the orders from the brain to the muscles to make them move (for more information, see the **General Introduction** section at the beginning of the book). If something happens to the nerves, the muscles don't work the way they are supposed to and actually get smaller. Without nerves telling them what to do, the muscles don't do much of anything important, and that means you are weak. So what kinds of things can hurt the nerves? Well, sometimes the immune system can attack the nerves by mistake. When this happens, we call it Guillain-Barré syndrome. For more information about the immune system and what can go wrong see the Chapter: **OTHER NERVOUS SYSTEM PROBLEMS**

One of the most common reasons that the nerves don't work right is that they aren't made right. As you get bigger, the nerves just can't keep up with everything they have to do. If the problem is just a little one, then the nerves don't start having problems until you are old. But if the mistake is a bad one, the nerves can have a lot of trouble early, like when you're a kid. You can also inherit bad wires from either your father or your mother–or maybe both (genes, again!). One of the most common diseases of the nerves that can be inherited is called Charcot-Marie-Tooth disease.

Now for the Muscles

Sometimes people have muscles that don't work right. These diseases are called myopathies or dystrophies. One is called Duchenne muscular dystrophy. And people who have bad muscles can look very much like people with bad nerves. Most of the tests are about the same too. Sometimes other things can happen to the muscles–like medicines and drugs can hurt the muscles, or sometimes the immune warriors can hurt the muscles (polymyositis).

How Can a Doctor Tell if Your Nerves or Muscles Are Messed Up?

There are some blood tests that are very special and done in special laboratories. Sometimes these tests can tell if you got your bad wires from your mom or dad.

Other important tests are called the EMG (electromyography) and NCV (nerve conduction velocity), which are done at the same time. They are really not so bad–see the person in the picture is smiling!

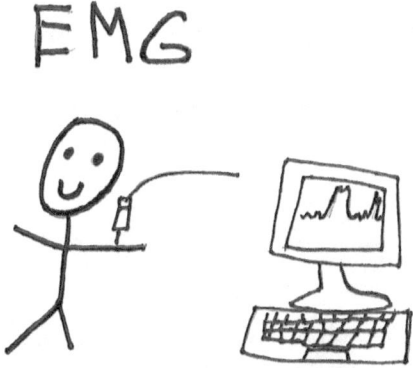

This is a test to see how well the nerves and muscles are working.

This test is in two parts.

The first part looks at how well your nerves carry electricity. Remember how your nerves carry electricity just like the wires in the wall? Well, we can test how well your nerves carry electricity by giving you a little signal (sort of like sticking your finger in a light socket–But don't do this at home!) and then measuring how much electricity moves down your arm (or leg) and how fast. The second part of the test listens in on the conversation between your muscles and nerves. You know, they do talk to each other all day long. The nerve tells the muscle what to do, and the muscles ask the nerve if they did it right. Well, what do you do when you get sick? You sometimes cry and complain, don't you? Well, your nerves and muscles can also cry and complain when they are sick. And there are special doctors who can listen to this talk between the muscles and the nerves and understand what they are saying. Then they can tell if it's the nerves or muscles (or both) that are unhappy and what's wrong. But because nerves and muscles don't talk very loudly, the doctor has to put a tiny microphone into your muscle. The microphone is in a tiny pin, and then you'll be able to hear your muscles and nerves too!

Finally, in some cases, if that doesn't give us the answer, we might have to take a piece of muscle or nerve and look at it under the microscope. And that may mean a small operation. But because of the EMG, we don't have to do that nearly as much as we used to.

Can We Fix It?

That depends on what's wrong. If the muscles or nerves are injured because of drugs or other things, these can sometimes be fixed. But if you have muscles or nerves that might have been designed wrong, then there is not much doctors can do. Some of the diseases mean that you just get weaker and weaker over time until you need a wheelchair. Those can be pretty hard. But there is a wonderful group of people called physical therapists who can help your muscles stay as strong as possible and keep you as active as possible. Besides, there are a lot of fun things you can do, even from a wheelchair!

Myth

A weak body does not mean a weak mind!

Voices of the Kids

Below are essays written by two children with weakness: Keri and Robert.

Meet Keri

In 2000 (Keri was nine when she wrote her first essay). Keri was born with nerves that don't work as well as they are supposed to. That means the muscles don't get the signals from the nerves, so they are not sure what to do. When that happens, your arms and legs are weak. If that happens before you are born, you don't move around as much in your mom's womb, so your arms and legs can get stuck in a funny position and not develop right. That is one reason a person like Keri has clubfeet (when the feet develop and look like a club instead of being flat).

In 2014 As you can tell from her follow-up essay, Keri has grown into a very articulate (good with words) college graduate. She didn't let the problem with her nerves get her down as a child—and doesn't as an adult.

In 2000

> My name is Keri. I'm 9 years old and in the third grade and I make straight A's. I live at home with my Dad, Mom and one brother named Matt. I also have two other brothers named Jeremy and Blair. And one niece named Kylie.
>
> When I was born I had clubfeet. When I was 4 months old I had surgery and again at 6

months old. I sometimes have pain in my legs and feet because of this, I'll have another surgery when I'm about 16 years old.

I have a bigger problem though. I have median nerve damage in both arms [the median nerve is the nerve that makes your first three fingers move and brings back feelings from those fingers to the brain]. I can't feel in my hands except for one finger, my ring finger. It is very aggravating to have this. It makes my arms and hands hurt all the time. I can't feel what's in my hands, or what I am holding. To pick things up, I have to use my pinky and ring finger. Sometimes I cut myself or burn myself and don't even know it.

The first time it was noticed, I was at my Grandparent's house. My Grandpaw noticed how I was picking things up and told my mom.

My Dad and Mom took me to the doctor. He said we had to go to a big city to have some tests done. They took some rods and stuck them through me to see if my nerves would move. I would have to move my fingers and hands around while they tested me.

That's when they found out nothing could be done about this. Now I see a neurologist who sends me to therapy and is going to try different things before I have to do another annoying test.

I can do anything anyone else can do but in different ways because that's the way God made me!

In 2014

My name is Keri. I am 23-years-old and a recent college graduate as of May 2014.

Because I was born with median nerve damage in both of my arms, I have learned to do things differently in order to accommodate the loss of feeling that I have in my hands and fingers. The issues that I have with my hands do not typically bother me, however, I do have difficulty handling or picking up small objects. Because of this, I often drop what I am holding and have trouble with such things as the clasp on a necklace or small buttons on a shirt. I take more time to pick up small objects, and to do so, I use my last two fingers as these are the fingers in which I have the most sensation. I sometimes accidently cut or burn my hands or fingers without noticing doing so. Because of this condition, I frequently experience numbness, weakness, and tingling in my arms and hands. Though this can be frustrating and difficult at times, I know no difference and have been able to adjust my ways of doing anything that I need.

As a child, I completed a nerve conduction study which told my doctor what was causing the lack of sensation in my hands as well as the extent of the issue. After having this test done, my parents were told that though surgery was possible, there would be risks along with an uncertain outcome. My parents decided that it would be best not to proceed. Because this condition does not hinder my ability to function normally, I do not feel that any treatment is necessary for me at this time.

When I wrote my last essay at 9-years-old, I had more difficulties with the median nerve damage in my arms than I did with my club feet. Today, the opposite is true. Though I can walk, I often have pain in my feet and legs. The physical deformities associated with club feet affect both my walking and ability to fit into some shoes. Along with the corrective surgeries that I had on my feet as an infant, I also had another surgery on my left foot about 3 years ago. In the future, I can expect to have additional surgeries on my feet and possibly on my knees and hips as well. These surgeries will help to relieve discomfort, correct deformities, and ensure my ability to continue to walk.

I feel about these conditions as I did when I was 9-years-old. These problems do not change who I am. I may do things differently, but I can do anything else can. These issues with my hands and feet do not hold me back.

Meet Robert

In 2000 (Robert was ten when he wrote his first essay). All his life, Robert would have times when he had trouble moving. After he had been sitting for a while or sleeping, he wouldn't be able to move at all. It usually got better after about fifteen minutes, especially if there was someone there to help him get started–sort of like pushing a car to get it running after you have let the battery run down. Finally, as he got bigger, it got harder for his mom to pick him up and walk him around until he got moving on his own, so she brought him to a neurologist.

Robert has inherited a disease called myotonia congenita. This is one of a group called ion channelopathies. That word looks complicated, but it really isn't. Remember how the nerves and muscles use electricity to talk to each other? How does the electricity get from the nerves to the muscles? It has to pass through special gates (ions) at the end of the nerve and into the muscles through special areas called channels.

Well, when people inherit a problem with the gates or the channels, bad things can happen. If there aren't enough gates or they don't work properly, the nerve sends electricity down to its tip. But there aren't enough gates to open, and so not enough electricity can get out! So the muscles don't get enough electricity to make them move. To finally make things go, the nerve has to send a lot of electricity down, because the few gates have to stay open for a really long time before enough electricity makes it to the muscles to get them moving.

That's why it takes Robert a while to get going. Think of it like your dad having to pull the starter rope on the lawn mower a whole lot of times before it finally starts! But because the muscles aren't working as well as they know they should, they try to make more of themselves to help out–which is why Robert looks really, really buffed, girls!

In 2014 Robert is doing terrific! His short report from 2014 makes it seem like his condition is just a part (and a minor part at that) of his life.

In 2000

My Story

By Robert

Once I was a little baby and my mother says I was so cute. She knew something was not quite right, because sometimes I could not walk or turn over. It was mostly at night and after a car ride.

I do not remember back then, but I'd like to tell you about how it feels now to have Myotonia congenita. It feels tight. You cannot move your muscles. You freeze.

When I was 2 we went to the park and everyone got out to run to the swings, but I could not move. Mama got me out of the car seat, and boom I fell flat. In baby talk I told her I could not walk. She laid me in the grass.

It was really hard because everyone else was playing and having fun. I could see them but I could not get to them no matter how hard I tried. I pulled myself in the grass and finally got there.

That is when she really began to try and figure this out. Finally we came upon two neurologists. They told me what it was right away. Only I had to go to a hospital in another city. They put a needle in my muscles to hear them talk. Did you know muscles talk? They do, only my muscles don't talk clearly to each other. They give wrong messages and I guess this is why my muscles don't work right, they get bad signals.

I still go to my doctors, but guess what, there is no way to fix this problem. Too Bad! Huh!

But I've learned some things that make it happen less.

1. Do not sit still for a long time.

2. Do not go car riding for more than 30 minutes. Get out at least every 20 minutes and walk around.

3. If the muscles are frozen, try to walk or pull up on something. Move around.

4. Keep walking until it is gone. Even try to run.

5. Eat good food and drink lots of water.

If you wanted to be my friend here is how you can help.

1. Pass on and mind your own business. Sometimes I look funny, waving my arms,

and dragging my leg. I even fall flat on my face. Don't stare.

2. Don't worry, it does not hurt. I will get out of it.

3. If I need you, I will call for you.

4. Keep sharp table points away so if I fall, I won't get hurt.

Mostly I can play and run just like you and that is what I like to do, have fun. We can have lots of fun together. One day I want to fly an airplane. I saw a man in a wheelchair fly one.

By

Robert

In 2014

Fortunately my condition has not severely progressed, and I'm currently in school for computer information.

Lessons for Adults

It's very hard for me to come up with the lessons for this chapter because the kids have done such a nice job of it themselves. I really can't beat Robert's step-by-step instructions, which he has stated so clearly. However, I would like to point out that we must do a better job of educating the classmates as well as the patients. Both kids have stated how they hated to be teased for their disabilities. No child with a neuropathy or myopathy should ever be bullied for being too slow or too weak. It is my hope that this book will be used by teachers as a starting point for classroom discussions so that all children can be educated and understand. It is clearly time that we bring these disorders out of the closet and discuss them openly.

One important point for adults to remember is that some of the testing, particularly the EMG and NCV (nerve conduction velocity), can be uncomfortable. I never lie to the children and tell them that it won't hurt. Instead, I explain exactly what the tests are for and why it's so important that we do them. I remember giving the explanation to a four-year-old, and weeks later during the test, she surprised the technician by jumping on the table, crossing her arms over her chest, and stating quite emphatically, "Now they are going to shock me!" Needless to say, she tolerated the testing very well.

CEREBRAL PALSY

What Is It?

THE TERM "CEREBRAL palsy" can be pretty frightening. What it means simply is that there is muscle weakness due to a problem with the brain rather than the muscles or the nerves (see the previous section). Usually, the muscles are too tight and stiff and very difficult to use. It also means that we do not expect things to get worse. It can be very mild so that the only problem is that a person walks on their tiptoes–or really severe. These people can be in a wheelchair and find it hard to use their hands. Also, the muscles that make speech can be affected, which is why it can be hard to talk (and for other people to understand). Cerebral Palsy also means that it is there as a baby and doesn't get worse (clarification of the definition of cerebral palsy).

What Causes It?

There can be many reasons that the brain is injured enough to cause tight muscles. Head injuries can damage the part of the brain that makes the muscles move (so that's why it is so important to wear your helmet when you ride a bicycle or a seat belt when you are in the car). Going too long without air can damage the brain. This can occur if you are swimming alone and start to drown. Sometimes, if a blood vessel gets clogged, not enough blood can get to parts of the brain, and these parts can die. This is called a stroke. While it most often happens to old people, it can also happen to kids. Cerebral palsy happens if that part of the brain is not formed right or is damaged by a difficult birth. One of the most common causes is when a baby is born too soon.

Sometimes we can't figure out why somebody has cerebral palsy.

What Happens to the Brain of a Baby that Is Born before It's Supposed to Be?

Do you have any little brothers or sisters? If you do, then you know that a baby is supposed to grow inside the mother's womb for about nine months.

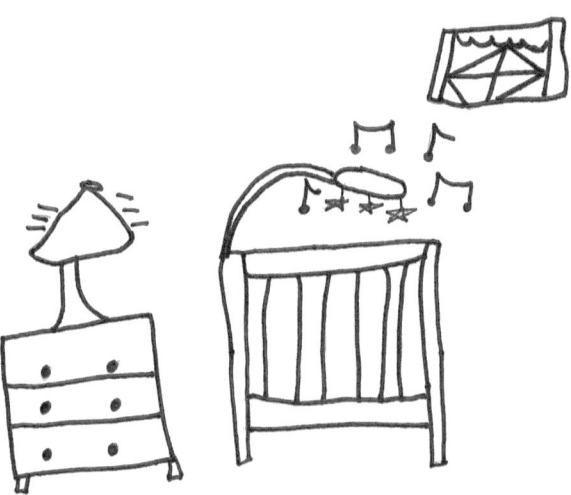

But sometimes things happen so that the baby is born too soon. It then has to do a lot of growing on the outside in special incubators until the baby is big enough to go home. Sometimes, these babies have brain problems, even though they got the best care possible, because the brain may not be ready to live outside. For example, some of the blood vessels (the tubes that carry blood to the brain) may not be strong enough, which can lead to leaking. However, doctors are getting much better at taking care of these babies, so this is happening less often.

How Do You Diagnose It?

The doctors talk to you and your family for a long time to decide if it sounds like cerebral palsy. They will probably do an MRI to look for any damage to the brain. Then they may do a bunch of other tests, depending on what they find.

How Can We Help?

Unfortunately, when brain cells die, they do not grow back. Sometimes other brain cells can take over the job of the brain cells that have died, and they can be taught to do the same things that the cells that have died were supposed to do. How do we teach new jobs to brain cells? We use different training methods. To retrain the brain cells that control the big muscles, we use physical therapy. This is to help with walking, sitting, running, hopping, and other activities like that. To retrain the brain cells that control the little muscles, we use occupational therapy, which helps with writing, using scissors, drawing, and all the other important things you do with your hands. Finally, the speech therapists help teach you to talk. Some therapy can really be fun like horseback riding, which helps with balance, and swimming, which helps make muscles stronger without having to stand on them.

Myths

Do you have cerebral palsy or know anyone with cerebral palsy? If you do, then you know how difficult it is to do the same activities that other kids can do. Sometimes it's hard to talk because speech can be slow and hard to understand, but that doesn't mean that you don't have some great ideas too! So if you know anyone with cerebral palsy, ask him or her if he or she might need some help with things occasionally. Also, take time to really talk with them and listen. If you have cerebral palsy, it's okay to ask for help sometimes. Kids with cerebral palsy can make great friends!

Even animals can get cerebral palsy. One of my patients had a kitten with cerebral palsy. He told me that the kitten's two front paws were very ugly because one paw had only three toes and the other paw was bent, but she was very happy and liked to play with him. Since she couldn't walk, she hopped like a rabbit. She was special, and he loved her dearly. Cerebral palsy did not stop this kitten from playing and loving her family, and it didn't stop her family from loving and playing with her.

Voices of the Kids

Below is an essay written by Megan, who has cerebral palsy.

Meet Megan

In 2000 (Megan was ten when she wrote her first essay). Megan is ten years old, and one of her favorite things to do is go shopping. She also has cerebral palsy. She is in a wheelchair and needs help with a lot of things that we take for granted. She has a hard time talking, so each word comes out slowly. But if you have patience, she has some interesting things to say!

In 2014 Megan is now twenty-three years old and an adult. Mom says, "Megan has a good quality of life living with her dad and I. Megan's physical health is fairly good. Besides the CP, which is pretty much involved, her biggest issue is spasms. She now has a [medicine] pump installed with quite a few issues. But it mostly helps to keep her spasms under control. Megan is a very social person and loved by all she meets."

In 2000

> Tight muscles are not good. It's not in a good way and I can't walk. Most kids can't walk that have CP.

Megan has been considering getting shots to help make the muscles less tight. When asked if she knew what this was, she replied, *"A shot to make me relax."* She then added, *"Shots are not the best thing in the world."* When she was asked if she still wanted to do it, she said, *"If it doesn't work, I don't need to go back. One day I may walk."*

In 2014

> I love my family and am somewhat OK with my life and condition. I will always have a desire to walk someday but until then I know I have to depend on other people for my care.

Lessons for Adults

Although treatments have greatly improved for cerebral palsy, we still have a long way to go. Currently, the options include medication, injections (of the paralytic botulinum toxin), and surgical implantation of a pump that provides medication directly to the brain. However, there are still many children who are totally disabled by CP.

When we see children with severe cerebral palsy, we often assume that their minds are as damaged as their bodies. But as you can see from reading the essay, that is not true. Megan has dreams, hopes, thoughts, and feelings, just like any other child. But because of their spasticity, each movement is restricted, and speech is slow and laborious. I remember seeing Megan for the first time. When we got to her medicines, I asked her if she preferred the liquid or the pill. She looked surprised, and her mother stated that that was the first time that a doctor talked to her, especially to ask her what she thought. And in fact, she had a decided preference. Megan told me that she needs to go up on her medicine and would like to do it with the nighttime dose.

So when meeting a child with severe CP for the first time, please determine if there is a mind inside before assuming there isn't.

NERVOUS SYSTEM PROBLEMS THAT AFFECT MOVEMENT

TICS AND TOURETTE'S SYNDROME

What Is a Tic?

WE JUST TALKED about diseases where movements are hard because the muscles are weak or the nerves or brain can't tell the muscles to move. But there are also diseases that cause movements we don't want! In neurology, we call these tics. A tic is a brief movement (motor tic) or noise (vocal tic) that you really didn't mean to do. The most common movement or motor tics include eye blinking and shoulder shrugging. Some of the common vocal tics are coughing, throat clearing, and sniffling. Sometimes vocal tics can be a habit of repeating words you hear or sometimes even saying bad words. However, saying a bad word after you dropped a rock on your bare foot is not a tic! Often, the tics will change over time, with some new ones starting while the old ones disappear.

If you have both motor tics and vocal tics for over a year and they seem to be getting more complex (like they started out with just eye blinking and now include eye blinking and shoulder shrugging), we call that Tourette's syndrome. Sometimes people with Tourette's syndrome also have problems with too much activity and not enough attention (see the previous section on ADHD/ADD) and obsessive-compulsive disorder. This is when you feel that you have to do something (compelled), like you have to touch every red tile in the room or walk a certain path or breathe in a certain way.

Most kids can control the tics a little bit, but they can build up then and "explode." Although tics can look funny, they are nothing to laugh about. People with tics are not doing them on purpose, and they can be uncomfortable. Sometimes, the person isn't even aware that he or she is having them. It is common that tics can get worse when a person is excited–even in a good way. Kids also complain that having tics all day can make their bodies sore.

Why Do I Have Tics?

Tics occur more often in boys than girls, and if your parents had them, you are more likely to have them. We don't really understand exactly what causes tics, but we think it has something to do with one of the chemicals that the brain uses. We think that the part of the brain that is supposed to keep these things from happening is a little lazy. For example, we have a tendency to think of the brain as being "off," and then when you want to do something, you turn that part of the brain "on"–sort of like a car that is turned off in the garage. However, the brain really doesn't work that way, because it's too slow. Think of how much time it takes for your parents to start the car: they have to put the key in the lock, turn the lock, and then let the car warm up before they can go anywhere. Instead, the brain is always "on" like a car that is left with the engine running in the driveway, but with the parking brake on to keep the car from moving. It's much faster to get the car moving if all you have to do is release the brakes. The brain also has "brakes" to keep you from doing something that you don't want to do.

But what happens if the parking brake slips while the car is running? The car starts to roll, right? Well, that's one way to think about tics. Your brain's brake slipped just a little bit, and these tics rolled out. Now think about a car with a slippery brake on a flat place–for example, Louisiana. It's pretty flat there, so chances are the car won't roll too far if the parking brake slips. Imagine that same car in the mountains or San Francisco, where the roads are very steep.

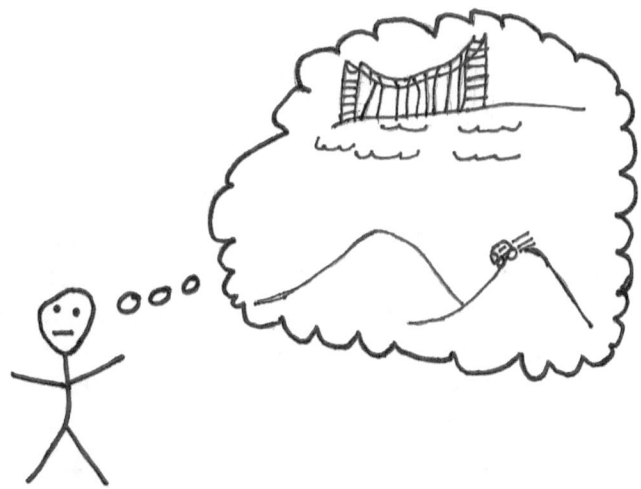

If that parking brake slips there, that car is going to roll pretty far and fast! For people with tics, being calm is like being on a flat road in Louisiana, but being nervous is like moving to the mountains or San Francisco!

I did have one child tell me that he felt like there was a ghost inside his head that makes the parking brake not work.

How Does the Doctor Decide if You Have Tics?

Most of the time, the doctor can tell if you have tics by talking with you and seeing the tics. Sometimes they may want to do some tests to make sure that there is not a more severe problem causing the movements. So they may do an EEG (to see if seizures are causing the tics), an MRI (to make sure there is not a tumor causing problems), and some blood or urine tests (for a description of the EEG and MRI, see the **General Introduction** section). If all these tests are negative and the doctor thinks they look like tics, he or she will tell you that is what you have.

Can We Treat Them?

The good news is that tics usually get better after you get older. They don't mean you have a horrible brain disease! So the best treatment is education (make sure people, especially teachers, realize what they are) and benign neglect (which means to ignore them). The more attention you pay to them, the worse they get (being nervous is like being in the mountains, remember?). Things that make tics worse include caffeine (sorry, no more Mountain Dew), some of the medicines that kids take to help with ADHD, and stress. To have the teacher call attention to the tics is *not* a good thing. There are some medicines around, but they don't work all that well and can have some bad side effects. So the best thing to do is relax: your brain is a good one, so don't offer to trade it!

Myths

Do you know who Samuel Johnson is? He was a very famous, smart person who invented the dictionary. I bet you have heard of Mozart, the incredibly talented musician that they made a movie about. (Go ask your mother to rent the movie *Amadeus*.) So why do I mention these guys? Well, some neurologists believe that they had Tourette's syndrome too! And Dr. Oliver Sacks, one of the most famous neurologists of our time, believes that Tourette's syndrome is what made them so creative.

So, although it may seem like it, these kids are not doing this to annoy you. They are not making "silly faces" or "rude noises." And it's not funny. So please don't laugh or tease someone with tics. If you have tics, please try to understand when someone asks why you are doing what you are doing. Be patient and take time to teach the person asking all about tics. After all, if they didn't want to know, they wouldn't have asked! That way, they can teach someone else!

Lessons for Adults

Tics are best treated with education and benign neglect. While there are medications available, they are less than miraculous in their efficacy and have a number of side effects. Many kids have told me that they find the tics less of a problem once they understand what tics are. One of my patients actually gave a presentation to his elementary class about tics so kids would understand him better and stop asking questions.

Adults, especially teachers, need to be able to recognize tics. Too often, the children are castigated for a behavior that they may be unaware that they are doing. When brought to the child's attention, they may be able to control the tics for a brief period of time; then, while concentrating on other things, the tics return. If unaware that this is a movement disorder, the teacher may again attempt discipline. This only increases the child's stress, which leads to more tics. If an adult finds the behavior annoying, he or she may gently remind the child. However, it must be recognized that during times of stress, the tics will increase, and this must be anticipated. Often, attempts to control the tics during the day will lead to an explosion of activity when the child returns home and relaxes. ADHD and tics often go hand in hand. The need for stimulant medication, which can make tics worse, must be assessed carefully. If the child with ADHD or ADD is truly in danger of failing in school, stimulant medication may be necessary, but the kids (and parents and teachers) need to understand that tics may be exacerbated so everyone can be prepared.

I am always surprised at how well the kids do after some reassurance. I always encourage them to take control of their lives and do something positive. For example, when one patient mentioned his dream of living on an island where everyone was just like him, I suggested he start a support group.

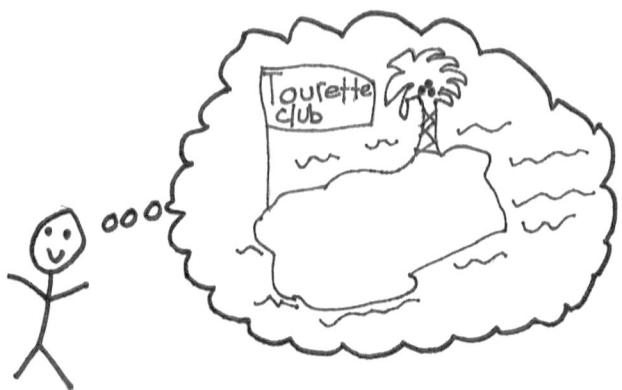

He left the visit planning to use his dad's computer to print notices about his "Tourette Club." We, as doctors and parents, shouldn't do this for the kids. Instead, it would be better to encourage the kids to do it for themselves.

MORE MOVEMENT DISORDERS
WHY IT CAN BE TOUGH TO KEEP ON MOVING

IF YOU'VE READ the other parts of this book, then you already know some reasons why people may have trouble moving. Sometimes it's because they are weak. People can be weak because either their nerves and muscles aren't very good, or the brain isn't very good at telling the nerves and muscles what to do. In the chapter before this one, we talked about problems kids had when they moved too much. In this chapter, we are going to talk about other reasons that some kids have trouble moving.

Friedreich's Ataxia (FA)

How do you know where to move? Well, first, you have to know where you are. That very important sensation is called joint position sense. I want you to try something for me. Stick your right hand out in front of you. Now close your eyes. With your other hand, point to the one out in front of you. I bet you know exactly where that right hand is, even if you can't see it. That is joint position sense. It is also why you don't have to watch your feet when you walk, because your brain knows where your feet are, most of the time anyway. If you have Friedreich's ataxia, the brain doesn't receive that information, and it's much harder to walk around, especially at night when it's dark and you can't see where your feet are. Since you can't watch your hands and your feet at the same time, it's hard to walk and do anything with your hands. Hands and feet that don't know where they are actually make continuous movements trying to "find themselves." So these extra movements can be a problem too. Unfortunately, we are not very good about fixing this problem, and it gets worse the older you are.

Parkinson's Disease

Do you have a grandparent whose hands shake (tremors) or who seems to move very slowly? Do they have trouble "getting their motor started"? Maybe they have Parkinson's disease. This is a disease that an older person (like your grandparents) gets and happens when the part of the brain that controls movement starts to break down. When this happens, parts of you move too much (like the hands shaking a lot), and other parts can't move fast enough (like legs in walking).

Although mostly older people get it, doctors know that young people can get it too. Michael J. Fox has it, and he's pretty young. It made it hard for him to act, and he had to quit his TV show, *Spin City*. But did you know there is a kind of Parkinson's disease that kids can get too? They don't usually get the shakes, but it can be very hard for them to move anything. Their muscles feel really rigid, and they get "frozen." Luckily, although we can't fix the part of the brain that isn't working right, we can give medicine that helps a lot.

Voices of the Kids

Below are essays written by two children with trouble with moving due to Friedreich's ataxia (Aaron) and juvenile Parkinson's disease (Brittani).

Meet Aaron

In 2000 (Aaron was thirteen when he wrote his essay). Aaron is really smart; he is really cute (although he already has a girlfriend). He likes to get in trouble, and he has Friedreich's ataxia (FA). FA is inherited (you have to get one bad gene from your mom and one from your dad). Aaron wants to share his story with you.

In 2000

TORMENT

By Aaron S.

Aaron's Story

My name is Aaron S. and I am thirteen years old. I have brown eyes and black hair, pretty good looking. (Sorry, I have a girlfriend…) I like hunting and fishing with my dad, and I like music. I LOVE music. I have a great CD collection. I also enjoy video games. I am a pretty typical thirteen-year-old. Except for one thing. I have FA. That's Friedreich's Ataxia.

I think I am very normal, but some differences are that I tire easy, I can't write for long periods of time, and I'm a bit clumsy. Although I'm a pretty good drummer, I can't play them for a long time like I used to. That is because my nerves are slow and it's like they have a mind of their own. To keep up with the rest of my body they have to work harder, and I guess they get tired, too.

Some things I miss are playing different sports, like baseball. I was never on the All-Star team, but I was pretty darned good. But I knew I couldn't run the bases as fast as I needed to, and I couldn't catch a fly ball. I remember one time during a game I swung; I missed the ball and fell down. Everybody got a good laugh at the expense of my feelings.

I can't write because to stabilize the pencil I have to squeeze hard. This makes me use the muscles so hard they start to hurt. But I don't miss that much because it makes schoolwork easier. Someone else gets to do my writing for me!

The Torment

When my pediatrician couldn't figure out why my body wasn't working right, we ended up at a large medical center. That's when all the tests began. And tests, and tests, and tests. Then there was the toe twitch test. The doctors put electrodes in my foot and made my big toe twitch when they put an impulse on it. My toe jerked all over the place. They told me to relax, but it's hard to relax when your toe is twitching like crazy.

I did get one good laugh, when I had my MRI (magnetic resonance imaging). Here I was, standing by that big machine wondering what in the world they were going to do to me now. The nurse walked in and came close to me, when all of a sudden this paper clip flew out of her pocket and soared across the room. The MRI is magnetic, and the giant magnet just pulled that paper clip right out. They are probably still looking for that paper clip today somewhere in that room!

Lousy Labs

Then there was the blood work. Back at home the doctors started on the lab work. I was starting to think they were taking out a little too much blood! It seemed like they were filling up an oil drum with it! One time they took so much blood I almost passed out. The cardiologist had me wear a heart monitor for 24 hours and told me to do all the normal things I usually do. So I went to a friend's house and played the drums (like I normally do). I can imagine what the monitor tape sounded like during that time!

After my diagnosis, I had X-rays to check for scoliosis. On one visit after the X-rays she found out the machine didn't work and I had to come back and do it all over again. I didn't even get to miss school because it was on the weekend! Another time, the technician got very mad because I could not stand still for the X-ray. Hey, it wasn't my fault!

Getting the News

Finally, the doctors were able to put a name on my disorder. Years of tests really didn't prove anything; it was the blood work that answered the questions. My mom and dad were in the exam room, when the neurologist came in and started talking to them about the blood test results. While she was explaining things to them, I was more worried about what we were going to eat for lunch, because I didn't understand what she was saying. But my mom started crying and I didn't understand. I knew I had something, but I wanted to know what it was and what it would do to me.

The doctor started to talk about X's and O's. To me X's and O's are used in football for offense and defense. They didn't mean anything to me. I left the office feeling confused because I didn't understand what FA was. I wasn't scared. I didn't feel changed because I wasn't any different than before my first test. Hey,

I was in 6th grade and I didn't understand genetics. Later, when I learned more about FA from every doctor appointment, I began to realize why this happened to me.

By this time things started to get more difficult for me in school. It was harder to hold a pencil and climb the stairs. They let me start using the elevator. My PE teacher sure didn't help much. He expected me to run as fast as everyone else, and do all twenty push-ups and all ten pull-ups. I mean, that's hard enough for a normal kid to do, let alone me! But my friends and I got him back. We pulled plenty of pranks, like untying the tether ball ropes he had just set up, or kicking over the cones he used for the running exercises. That made me feel better!

My other teachers tried to help. They did what they were told, like oral testing so I wouldn't have to write, and let me be late for class when I had to cross campus from one class to another. Most of the other students were nice, but there were a few that were mean. But my friends and I got them back, just like the PE coach. This one kid just wasn't cool with me. So one day my friend and I took his shoes in the PE locker room and tied the laces together, then tossed them over the beams in the ceiling so he couldn't reach them. Now that is justice!

Well, public school wasn't cutting it, so in the fall of the 8th grade we tried private school. At first it was fun until the work began. I was on the flag football team and made new friends. But then, I started talking to my friends all the time and I started worrying less about my schoolwork. It was frustrating to do the written work because I always had to leave the room to get writing help. I just couldn't handle using a pencil or pen. So second semester, we started home schooling. In fact, I wrote this story as an English assignment. As of now, I like it because there is no frustration, and I can do my work better. I know my education is important, so I can go to college and study music.

MDA Camp

It's important to me to remember I am a kid. Not a kid with FA, but just a regular kid. The summer going into 8th grade I got a chance to be just that. I spent a week at an MDA [Muscular Dystrophy Association] camp with other kids who had just as hard a time at baseball as I did. And it felt AWESOME.

I rode a bus to Camp Bethany with other campers from the area. We settled into large cabins, where I shared a room with three other campers and the counselors. My counselor's name was Scott. He was a college student, so we hit it off right away. The other campers ranged from about eight years old to eighteen.

What a week! We swam, went fishing, did arts and crafts, played basketball and other sports, and lots of other activities. It was great to just play and not worry about how fast or how well I did something. I was just "me."

It was the week of the College Baseball World Series, and LSU and ULL were both playing. One of my friends was a Tennessee fan, and of course they were eliminated, so he wasn't too happy. But I was rooting for my teams, and we even took some "illegal" bets on the scores, using the fake money we earned at camp for different activities. I cleaned up! I went with LSU, which of course, won.

Lots of pranks were pulled that week, and I was in the middle of most of them. Not to get into a long story, but they included feathers and ceiling fans, water balloons, shaving crème, and the girls' cabins. Leaving your cabin during rest hour made you a fugitive to the camp master, Casey. Since Casey lived in my cabin it made it difficult to get away with sneaking out. I did get in trouble for that, but I got over it.

We earned camp money by reaching goals, like catching fish, crafts projects, carnival games, and swimming. I made lots of money on the dunking booth because I teamed up with a great pitcher. We spent our money at the camp store, where we could buy CD's, books, shirts, remote control cars, mugs, toys, and all sorts of stuff. I had a small fortune at the end of the week and went on a spending spree.

By the end of the week I felt so much better about myself. There were other people who feel the same way I do, who live the same way I do, and act the same. But there were also kids who had it much harder. Some had to wake up during the night to take medicine and shots, some were in wheelchairs, or had IV's and pumps. It made me feel lucky, for sure. I could get in the water and do what I wanted without my counselor being right there. I felt good about myself. I can't wait to go back next summer.

A Future With Friedrich's

My life has changed a lot in the last few years. Once I thought I wanted to be an NFL star or an architect. Now I know I will have to work with what I have. I know I have music talent, and for now I want to be a musician. I want to go to college. I guess I want to be in love.

I am going to have to work a lot harder to get there. I will have to have a lot of help with school, and it will be harder to find a job I can handle when I turn sixteen. I might get a lot more clumsy. I might end up in a wheelchair. No one knows that for sure. So I will have to prepare myself for whatever gets in my way.

I know scientists are learning new things every day that will help me with my ataxia. Who knows, five years from now I might be able to walk down the street without people turning their heads! I really am just like any other kid my age. I don't know what direction I will take but I'm excited to get there.

Meet Brittani

In 2000 (Brittani was thirteen when she wrote her first essay). Brittani has juvenile Parkinson's disease. It took her doctors a long time to figure it out because it doesn't happen very often in kids. But she was patient with the many doctors she had to see, and they finally got her on a medicine that really helped a lot.

In 2014 Brittani has had some major challenges in her life, as she describes in her second essay. However, she has achieved her goals of graduating from college and has a beautiful daughter. While she talks about some disappointment in having to change her major from early childhood education to general studies, I like to think that her willingness to share her story here means she is able to teach and help children.

In 2000

Unknown Torment

Hi, my name is Brittani. I am thirteen years old. I have hazel eyes, brown hair and very tall for a girl my age. I enjoy being with family and friends.

My torment started when I was in the eighth grade. My family noticed that I was off balance and had trouble walking and was always too tired to do any of the things I use to do. I was the lead person on our basketball team the years before and that year I could not keep up with the fast pace that basketball takes. Classmates noticed the way I walked and started teasing me by calling me a robot that made me sad. My mother decided it was time to go to our pediatrician for a check up to see what could be my problem. At his office he gave me a series of skill tests and did lab work on me and told us that there was something wrong but he did not know what it could be. He had his nurse make an appointment for me to see a neurologist. He said that something was wrong with the functioning of my brain and he needed me to see another doctor. A few days later I met my doctor. At her office she put me through just about the same skill test the other doctor had done and she also noticed that something was terribly wrong with me. She spoke with me one on one and to my parents and explained that in order to find out what was wrong she had to do a series of tests which included a CAT scan and blood work and she said if there was something wrong on the CAT scan we would have to leave for the hospital today. Everything was happening so fast and I was scared to find out what was wrong. After the test was completed they called me back in her office to explain the results, we didn't have to go to the hospital that day. From that visit many trips to doctor after doctor were to follow. She sent us to several doctors she thought would be able to find out my problem. I saw another doctor when he did my muscle biopsy. He spoke with my neurologist and asked her to try me on a medication, because he said it looked like a disease call Parkinson's. She started me on the medication and within a couple of days I could move around more like my old self. The doctors still don't know for sure if it's Parkinson's disease but the medication does wonders for me. If I don't take the medicine my feet feel like they are glued to the floor, my left leg drags, I get tired, and I start trembling. When I am feeling this way I just want to sleep. I can't do anything with my family and friends. I feel different than other teens and I really don't like telling them about my problem cause I am ashamed, I know this is not my fault, but it gets hard to cope with at times.

As for my family who have been very concerned about my illness and supportive of me I love them dearly. Traveling to and from the hospital to see doctors has been hard for them physically and financially. But they will do what everything it takes to find out what is my problem. My brother has a special place in my heart. He helps me do things that I can't when I am feeling tired. I thank my best friend Tracy for being there for me when I needed someone to talk to and just be myself. She knows all about my illness and it makes it easier for me to talk to her about the way I feel.

Last but not least I thank the Almighty God who has his angels watching over me 24-7.

To all who are suffering from unknown illness don't be scared just keep God in your heart at all times. I pray every day that they can find out what is wrong with me. When they do find out what is wrong I pray that it is something that can be cured. I want to have a normal life one day get married and have children.

In 2014

<u>My Present Life with YOPD</u> [Young Onset Parkinson's Disease]

Throughout all my struggles and tough times during my high school years, I graduated number five out of eighty six classmates. I received a TOPS scholarship, highest average in French, and a check for $300 from Guaranty Bank. I started college at LSUE in August 2003 to pursue my career as an Early Childhood Teacher or an Elementary teacher. I suffered from severe anxiety and panic attacks my first semester at LSUE. I drove back and forth from school at least three days a week. I went through my first semester okay even though I felt like people were always whispering and laughing at me. I guess that's just how judgmental some people were to me.

I stayed on campus in Bengal Village for the majority of my college years. I received my help from the Louisiana Rehabilitation Services in Lafayette, LA. I was blessed to have them pay for my college tuition, course books, and my resident monthly fee at Bengal Village. I had awesome grades in the majority of my courses. I had to repeat some of my Elementary and Early Childhood Math courses. I went to college during the Fall, Spring and Summer.

Sometime in October I met this wonderful, nice, and sweet guy that I thought was my promise prince. We dated and spent a lot of time together going to the movies, skating, eating out, clubs and etc. Well, I slipped up and got pregnant in January 2006. Our friends with benefits relationship continued even though my Psychologist warned me that I was seeing the relationship for how I wanted to see it. My parents were disappointed but they didn't know what to do because of my illness. My mom called my doctor, at the time to determine whether I should terminate the pregnancy or just go through it. I was high risk while I was pregnant due to PD. My doctor took me off as much medication as he could that would be harmful to my baby. I sat out of college the next couple of semesters.

In July 2007, I had my first DBS (deep brain Stimulation) surgery on the right side of my brain. It helped the first six months or so and then it began to tremendously affect my driving, mental state, and etc.

My second DBS was done in November of 2010 around Thanksgiving time. Throughout all my struggles and hurdles with this PD monster, I was able to graduate from ULL with my Bachelor's Degree in General Studies with a concentration in Behavioral Science. I am currently a single parent to my beautiful eight year old daughter named Briana. She is what keeps me in the fight with this horrible disease. My supportive family, church family, and friends have helped me out a great deal.

As for my medication treatments now, I take anywhere from eight to ten medications a day.

I have tried depression pills. I didn't notice much of a change. I have taken [a medicine] for my dyskinesia but it really didn't help me though. I have tried acupuncture and massage therapy the relief only last for about an hour or so. I suffer with excruciating and chronic pain in my back on a daily basis. I walk and stretch as much as I can when I'm in a good mood and full of energy. The best prescription for PD (Parkinson Disease) is WALKING.

Needless to say, I did go back to college to finish and get my Bachelor's Degree in Early Childhood Education. Next semester would be my last in which I would be student teaching. The pressure and stress started to destroy me quickly. My Math professor noticed a difference in my demeanor. She had a one on one talk with me as well as another one of my teacher was telling me negative stuff like she could not see me as a professional Reading teachers and that the stress with being a teacher would aggravate illness a lot more, but I love kids. I had to make a decision to change my major General Studies. This was a very devastating decision for me because I love teaching, working with, and helping students. I cried so much because my classmates were so good at helping me and checking me. I would not be graduating with them.

General Studies required only two classes for me to take for my last semester. I drove back and forth to UL two days a week. I passed both courses with a "B". I graduated December 19, 2009 from UL-Lafayette with my Bachelor's Degree in General Studies and a Minor in Behavioral Science. This was the happiest day of my life because my determination had finally paid off in a good way.

Lessons for Adults

Both of these kids faced and still face a future of progressive loss of function. There is no cure for what they have. Yet they consider themselves normal kids. Aaron, aside from his disease, was a typical teenager—having friends, getting into trouble, feuding with adults. Brittani had dreams she worked toward, had successes, and had problems just like we all do. They want out of life what we all want—happiness, love, and friendship. Most importantly, they don't see their future as one of loss but one of exciting possibilities, and they look forward to it eagerly.

But it distresses me that they can still feel ashamed by their disease. We need to do better in educating people that these kids are really no different than you or me. They don't want pity or special treatment—they just want to be kids.

OTHER NERVOUS SYSTEM PROBLEMS

Autoimmune Disorders, Brain Tumors, Degenerative Diseases of the Nervous System

AUTOIMMUNE DISEASE AND THE NERVOUS SYSTEM

WHEN YOUR BODY ATTACKS ITSELF (Guillain-Barré Syndrome, Transverse Myelitis, ADEM, Optic Neuritis, Multiple Sclerosis, CIDP)

What Is the Immune System?

THE IMMUNE SYSTEM is the part of the body that fights off infection. It is there to attack those horrible "bugs" that can make you sick with colds, the flu, sore throats, and earaches. Picture your body as a giant video game like in the picture below.

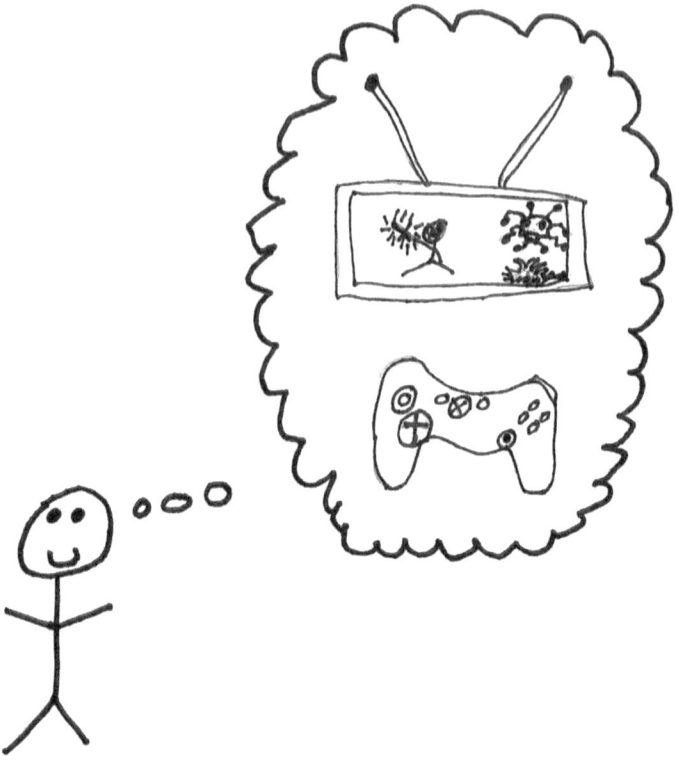

The horrible bugs have attacked, and the body must fight them off! So the immune system first gathers, determines just what kind of bugs they are, what weapons they have, and how to find them no matter where they try to hide. The immune system then creates a perfect warrior, especially designed to hunt down those evil bugs and destroy them (there is a different warrior for each type of bug). It then builds a factory where millions of these warriors can be made. The warriors are sent out to hunt up and destroy all the bad bugs. After the bad guys are all destroyed, the warriors are turned off, except for a very few who hang around in case the same bugs decide to come back. It's really important to turn off most of the warriors because a warrior without any enemies to fight becomes bored and can get into trouble.

So What Goes Wrong?

Since the immune system is so complicated, sometimes things can go wrong. Very rarely, the warriors sent out after the evil bugs have trouble telling the good guys from the bad guys because, occasionally, those clever bugs have learned to disguise themselves so they look like parts of the body. Sometimes the bugs end up disguising themselves to look like the brain, the nerves, or the muscles. When that happens, the warriors will get confused and attack the brain or the nerve or the muscles.

What Happens when the Brain or Nerves or Muscles Are Attacked?

If the warriors have attacked the brain, it can get harder to control your body, and you can do, say, and think things that aren't right. When this happens only once and you get sick only one time, it is called ADEM (acute demyelinating encephalomyelitis). When it happens more than once and you get sick more than once, it is called multiple sclerosis.

Sometimes the same thing can happen to the spinal cord, the big bundle of nerves that runs down your back. The nerves that go to your arms and legs are plugged into it. When the warriors attack here, nothing works well below where the problem is, and you might not be able to walk. What is embarrassing is that you can't always control your body, and you might have bathroom accidents when you don't want to. This is called transverse myelitis.

When other nerves are attacked, you can't move your arms or legs. Sometimes you can't breathe, and the doctors have to have a machine breathe for you. This is called Guillain-Barré syndrome. If it keeps happening, it's called CIDP (chronic inflammatory demyelinating polyneuropathy).

How Can Doctors Tell What's Wrong?

That depends on what part of the body is affected. For example, if it's the nerves or muscles, we do many of the same tests that are done for muscle and nerve problems (see the section of weakness or the **General Introduction** section). If the problem is in the brain, we will do an MRI to look for evidence of the warriors' battles. If you are having seizures, we will do an MRI. If the problem is with the spinal cord, we will take a picture of that. But the best test to see if the warriors are the problem is to capture some. Since they are wandering around your nervous system, that's where we have to go to get them. And the best place to look is in the fluid around you brain and nerves, called CSF (cerebral spinal fluid). It is very much like having blood taken out of your arm. We can then find these warriors and figure out what went wrong with them.

How Can We Fix It?

Luckily, the body can make new nerves and muscles, and the part of the brain that the warriors like to attack may be able to repair itself too. So all the doctors have to do is stop those confused warriors. There are two important ways to do that.

The first is to get rid of the warriors. Sometimes the doctors will give you a medicine that hunts up all these warriors and turns them off. Sometimes the doctors will hook you up to a blood washing machine and wash out all the bad warriors (plasmapheresis). Most of the time, those treatments are enough to get rid of all the problem-causing warriors.

But if the factory keeps making more warriors, then the doctors will use another medicine (steroids) to close down the factory. Once all the warriors are gone and the factory stops making more, the body can start to repair itself. Most patients get a lot better, but the brain and nerves are slow to heal, so it can take a long time. Since the repaired parts might not be as good as the old, there may be some things that you can't do as well as you could before. However, most kids end up almost as good as new.

Voices of the Kids

Below are essays written by Claudia and Shanda, two children with autoimmune diseases.

Meet Claudia

In 2000 (Claudia was eleven when she wrote her first essay). Claudia has been diagnosed with an autoimmune disease called multiple sclerosis and is on a medicine, which she will probably have to take for the rest of her life. That's a real pain because it's a shot. Since multiple sclerosis is very rare in children, it took a long time for her doctors to figure out what was wrong with her. Luckily, once they did and got her on the right medicine, she has done very well!

In 2014 She has done extremely well as she tells us herself!

In 2000

M.S. and me

by Claudia

age: 11

Hi! My name is Claudia. I like to skate, dance and ride 4-wheelers and I hope someday to be a pediatrician. Oh and I have a disease called multiple sclerosis (ms) and I would like to tell you about it.

It all started happening in February 1998 around my birthday; by the way my birthday is February 24th. I was always feeling tired and sleepy. My mom and dad were very worried about me. All I wanted to do was sleep. I never wanted to play or eat or go anywhere. My teacher was also concerned because I was falling asleep at school a lot. I was also complaining with my eye hurting. So my mom and dad decided to take me to the doctor. When we told him my symptoms he began to check me out. He had the nurse to draw some blood, which I hated, but it only hurt a little bit and then he checked my eyes. Come to find out I had gone blind in my right eye and did not even realize it. The doctor said that was because my other eye automatically took over and helped out and I didn't even know it. The next thing we did was that doctor sent me to an eye specialist. There they did all sorts of tests and said my eyes were fine; it was something else causing the problem. From there it all started I stayed in and out of the hospital (a whole bunch!).

One day me, mom and some family just got done shopping in Branson, Missouri when I got a headache and starting to things. When we got home I went blank. My mom, nanny and my sister got scared. They rushed me to an airplane so my doctor at home could take a look at me. On our way to the airport my Uncle Daryl was trying to make me blink but I wouldn't. It was like I was trying to get out but I couldn't. I was scared that I wouldn't wake and I would die. But I'm still here, obviously, or I wouldn't be telling you this story. When we got to the hospital, the doctors told me that I had a seizure. Here I went again in the hospital. They did lots of tests on me. I had MRI's that is an x-ray of your brain. It doesn't hurt really, you just have to have a small IV in your arm so your brain will show up better and it is very loud! I also had some spinal taps. That is when the doctor puts a tube in your back and draws fluid off of your spine. I didn't feel any of that even though I was awake because they give you medicine to make you feel silly and the best part is my mom and dad got to be there with me through all these tests.

Well after many months of being in and out of the hospital and lots of tests the doctors told me I had a disease called multiple sclerosis. That is a disease that affects your brain and nervous system. But it's okay. I am on a medicine I have to get shots three times a week. That's kind of yucky but hey, it keeps all my M.S. symptoms under control so it's worth the trouble. My big sister is a nurse and she gives them to me so it's okay. My neurologist lets me talk about things that are bothering me and never keeps anything from me. Sometimes when I tell people I have M.S. it scares them but I just let them know hey!, I'm not scared-I just take it one day at a time.

In 2014

You inspired me to not only write an essay but I wrote a book as well! And wrote it, then rewrote it. 14 years later it's still a work in progress, I can't seem to end it. (This is probably because my story isn't through). But if there is one lesson I learned from you, it is that I have no limits and M.S. is not a barrier.

Meet Shanda

In 2000 (Shanda was thirteen when she wrote her first essay). Shanda's problem began with unusual hiccups that wouldn't go away. They were very disruptive, making it hard for her to sleep, breathe, and concentrate. They even occurred while she was sleeping. She saw many doctors who tried her on many different medications. None of them worked. All the tests that were done were normal, so the doctors couldn't tell her what was wrong or how to fix it. She had to stop her activities because the hiccups made it hard for her to breathe. She missed so much school that she had to switch to homeschooling. Finally, her doctors thought that maybe this was a neurological problem caused by her immune system. Maybe Shanda had an infection that triggered the immune system to get overexcited, so her doctors gave her steroids to shut down the factory. Luckily, the hiccups went away!

In 2000

Hi, my name is Shanda. I'm thirteen years old. I've got strawberry blonde hair and brown eyes. I've got an infection, which nobody knows what it is.

It all started on a Tuesday morning in gym class right when I was going to track practice. My friends said it looked like I had the hic-ups, but my throat was making a very funny movement. Then I went to get some water to get rid of what I thought was the hic-ups, but it just didn't stop. I went to the office to see what I should do, but they didn't know, so I got on the bus thinking they would go away the next day. But I was wrong.

Within two days I was just sitting on the couch doing my homework when my mom noticed it. She asked me if I was okay, and I said no, so she went back in her room, and woke my dad up, and took me to the closest hospital to see what was wrong. But they didn't do anything. So the third time they took me to the big hospital, then they did more blood tests, more x-rays, more cat scans, and still couldn't find anything wrong.

I went to my regular doctor and he looked down my throat but he didn't know how to treat it. So he recommended me to an ears, nose, and throat doctor and he looked down my throat with a scope. What he said was that my little palate in the back of my throat was sticking to the back of my throat. He said that the only reason I was making the funny movement was because I was trying to keep it open. He did not know what to do so he recommended me to a big medical center and another ENT doctor. She stuck another scope down my throat, but she recorded it. Then she sent me to the 7th floor to see a neurologist.

He scheduled a MRI the next day. After that, he ordered for me to get blood work done, and gave me a prescription of medicine for the tic, and told my parents to call him if anything went wrong with the medicine and to come back in two weeks if anything did not work out. The second time back he ordered for me to get a chest x-ray to see if my diaphragm was spasming and got more blood work done, and gave me another thing of medicine to try and told me to come back in two weeks. When I came back I got an IV started and went down to get a spinal tap done. After that I came back and got another chest x-ray and x-rays of my throat, and he gave me more medicine, and told me the same thing. Then when I came back he took me to a conference where they all started thinking of things to do, and the next day I had to get more blood work, more cat scans, and a MRI. Then they gave me another medicine. They also ordered me to get this thing done of my brain waves to see if I did it in my sleep or whatever it was for.

When I came home for that two weeks I caught a cold and had to go to my regular doctor. She ordered for me to go to a sleep center to see if I did it in my sleep and a cat scan. Then after that I went back to my neurologist who told me and my parents that he was going to give me more bottle of medicine and if it did not work he was going to put me in the hospital for a few days with IVIG. Then within a few days of taking the medicine I started to break out like I did with everything else, and my parents called the doctor. He said to bring me in, and he was going to admit me.

When I got admitted I saw some Indian doctor and another bunch of doctors who decided to try steroids. While I was in there they did all kinds of tests like blood test, chest x-rays and something else. Then after that when I was about to go home I had to get an MRI.

After that, a neurologist came up and started talking to me, and to tell me what they figured was wrong with me. I mean I had the best doctors trying to learn and understand my problems. They all tried so much and finally found something out that was my problem. Now that I'm OK I can say I really had a lot of people to thank for helping me through all of the tests and this annoying problem I had. If somebody out there has this problem and you think you're the only one, just remember I'm out there with it too.

In 2014

My name is Shanda, I'm now 27 years old. When I was younger around 13 years of age

I had gotten sick. I had what was believed to be a severe case of the hiccups. But come to find out I had an infection in my body that attached itself to my throat causing me to make a noise that resembled having hiccups. They hospitalized me for a few days pumping me full of antibiotics and steroids. The steroids were the only thing to stop it.

Once they finally figured out the only thing that would work and stop the infection was steroids, my parents finally knew that if this was to happen again they would know how to treat it.

This bizarre incident happened one more time; this time I was either 15 or 17 at the time, my parents took me to the ER and everyone there didn't know what to do. My dad told my nurse that it had happened before and what they did to help me. So they hooked me up to an IV, gave me antibiotics and steroids and it went away. They sent me home with the same antibiotics and steroids. It has not happened or come back in years. I'm now living a happy and healthy life.

Lessons for Adults

The striking thing about these autoimmune disorders is the rapidity with which they can progress. With Guillain-Barré and transverse myelitis, kids can lose the ability to move their legs within hours. Claudia also mentions how fast her symptoms came on. I have seen children with Guillain-Barré syndrome go from completely normal to ventilator dependent in a matter of hours. When a child experiences a loss of neurologic function (walking, breathing, involuntary movements) that comes on acutely, the best place to take them is an emergency room. Walk-in clinics are oftentimes not set up to handle these cases. While not rare, they are uncommon enough that these clinics might not see enough of them to become familiar with them. Early diagnosis is crucial not only to prevent death from impaired respiratory dysfunction but also because there are treatments available. The sooner these treatments are started, the better the course of the disease. And in some situations, like Shanda's, the etiology may be elusive, requiring a leap of faith by both the patient and physician.

Finally, physicians can be intimidating. We toss around words like "autoimmune," "plasmapheresis," "ADEM," etc. Kids, as well as their parents, can end up more confused after a doctor's visit then before it. I use the video-game explanation to make the disease more understandable to the children who have it. However, I have found that many parents appreciate the lack of "doctorese."

BRAIN TUMORS

What Is a Brain Tumor?

WELL, THE FIRST part is pretty easy. It's a tumor that is in your brain. Now on to the second part–what is a tumor? Well, that is a little more difficult. Your body is made up of a gazillion cells that all work together. When all the cells in one area are about the same and do the same job, we call it an organ (like your kidney, which is made up of cells whose job it is to wash your blood). The groups of cells we are most interested in are the ones that make up your brain. These cells are all located in your head, and their job is to keep the body working in an organized manner and have fun doing it.

Each cell can divide and make two cells, and two cells can make four cells and so on. This is important because this is how you grow so you don't stay the size of a baby forever, and it is how an organ can heal itself after it gets hurt. There are very important signals that tell the cell when to divide and make more cells and when not to. A tumor forms when a group of cells decide they don't want to listen to these signals anymore, and they are going to continue to grow. Because they are making more cells so fast, all these cells start to pile up, and your body stops working right.

So What's the Problem?

These tumor cells are so busy making more cells that they can't do their job properly. Even worse, they have a tendency to get in the way of the cells that are trying to do their jobs. Also, there is only so much room in your head, since your skull is hard and can't get bigger very fast. So when the tumor cells in the brain grow too much, they get too big for the space and start pushing on the brain. This pressure is why you can have headaches. And everybody is worried because if we can't get rid of every last cell, they can come back.

How Do We Find Them?

Doctors can find tumors using pictures like CTs and MRIs. Sometimes we have to do special pictures to help better decide what kind of tumor it is. Sometimes, loose tumor cells can also be seen under a microscope, so we collect fluid from around your brain to catch any of the abnormal cells. Knowing what kind of tumor it is becomes very important when the doctors have to decide what is the best way to kill them and cure you.

So What Can We Do to Make Tumors Go Away?

The most important first step is to *get those guys out of there!* That's why the doctor often has to operate, and he has to shave your head so he can see what he's doing. For some tumors that is enough because all the tumor cells stay in the same place, so they are easy to find and take out. But some tumors have cells that like to travel to other parts of the brain and your body. So the doctors have to send out the marines to hunt these cells down and kill them. There are two ways to do that. To kill the wandering cells in the brain, we nuke 'em! We give high levels of radiation just to the brain and spinal cord. After that, we give chemotherapy. These are very powerful drugs that can kill the tumor cells and also kill the tumor cells that wander to other parts of the body. Since they make the rest of the body sick, your hair falls out, you bleed more easily and can get infections. But a lot of times, these things work and the brain tumor is defeated!

What Happens After?

Even if we can find all the tumor cells and make them go away, most often, the brain is not as good as it used to be, so it doesn't work as well. You will probably have more trouble thinking than you did before. But we have special people that can help make things easier. And you should be proud! You've fought a really tough battle, and *you won*!

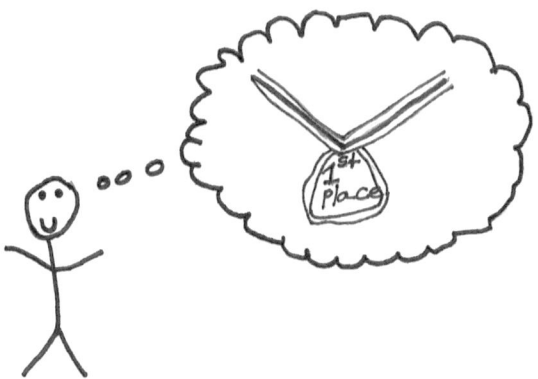

Voices of the Kids

Below is an essay written by Kirkland, who experienced two brain tumors.

Meet Kirkland "F"

In 2000 (Kirkland was sixteen when he wrote his first essay). Kirkland has had significant problems with two brain tumors, and because of these tumors, he has suffered with headaches. Yet even with everything that F has been through, he still remains optimistic about life and his future.

In 2014 Kirkland was happy to share his progress when I approached him fourteen years later. And he is still as optimistic as he always was.

2000: HOW I SURVIVED TWO BRAIN TUMORS BY KIRKLAND

Hi, my name is Kirkland, and I am a sixteen year old Junior in High School. I am a Christian, and I have survived two brain tumors, by the grace of God. All my friends and doctors call me "F" or "Fortune", because when I was younger, I used to love the Wheel of Fortune television show, and because I feel very fortunate. My story with brain tumors started back in December, 1988. I was four and a student in Headstart. When my mother would wake me up to go to school, I would have severe headaches, and go back to sleep for about four hours.

So, my mother took me our family doctor, but he couldn't find anything wrong with me. My mother remembers that I didn't feel normal during those holidays. All I wanted for Christmas was a Playschool flashlight. I still have it, and it is still working. We use it when the lights go out.

After the holidays, I went back to school, but was tired all the time. My mother noticed that my left eye was crossing, so, she took me back to my doctor, and he ordered a CAT scan on my head. The next day he called my mother to his office. He had already made plans for us to go to a big medical center, because it seemed I had a brain tumor.

The neurologist was waiting for us. Later we met the neurosurgeon. After taking many tests, including an MRI, he found out that I had fluid around my brain. So, he put a shunt in my head to drain the fluid. A shunt is a long, thin tube that is threaded under the skin to another part of the body, usually the abdomen. It works like a drainpipe. I still have the same shunt today. I had lost most of the sight in my left eye by then.

I was in surgery for twelve hours. The tumor was removed successfully. It was a Pineal Teratomal tumor. These tumors occur in the pineal gland, a tiny organ near the center of the brain. It can grow slowly or fast. The pineal section of the brain is very difficult to reach, and these tumors are very difficult to remove. The tumor was benign.

Then, it all started over again! I was going to the medical center every six months for check-ups and MRIs. In the summer of 1995 I began getting weak and tired, and did not want to go outside to play. My left side was getting weaker. My mother called my neurologist in September. She ordered another MRI and other tests, including a spinal tap. I had another brain tumor! Naturally, I was shocked and upset. This new tumor was a germ cell tumor, which is a tumor that begins in the cells that create sperm or eggs. The tumor can occur anywhere in the body and can be either benign or malignant.

So, I got two more doctors: a pediatric hematologist and an oncologist put me in the hospital for a few days. By then, I was having a hard time walking, and my left side was hurting, as well as my arm and leg. The doctors decided they couldn't do surgery, as it would be too risky and jeopardize the sight in my good eye. My doctors explained to me that if she stuck a straw up my nose, where it would stop, that was where my tumor was. So, how would they treat me if they couldn't do surgery?

The doctors decided that it would be best to treat me with radiation to my head and spine. They wanted to make sure that the germ cells didn't travel to my spine. The radiation treatments shrunk the tumor but because of the treatments, I had lost all of my hair. While I had been in the hospital, the pediatric social worker sent my name to the Make a Wish Foundation. In May, they got in touch with me to see what my wish was. I told them I would like to visit Disney World in Florida. So, during the last week of May, my mother, my brother and I went to Disney World on the airplane. We had Make a Wish buttons, and I had a Make a Wish cap that identified us, so we didn't have to wait in those long, long lines. We got to skip to the front of all the lines! That was fun. Although it was very hot there, we had a great time and took many pictures and made a video.

I have been going to Camp Rap-A-Hope every summer for a week since 1997. It is a Children's Oncology Camp. Nurse Judy is a pediatric oncology nurse at my hospital, and she and the Childlife Worker, Renee, each take a van full of kids to camp, then go back and get them. I've met some wonderful people at camp, and keep in touch with some of them.

I had a bone density test earlier this year that showed that I have the bones of a sixty-year-old. Also, you should see my gray hair that goes with my old bones! I have osteoporosis from the years of taking steroids. I have to be careful not to fall, because this could break my bones. I take extra calcium, but I don't drink milk because I just don't like it.

My oncologist tells me often that I'm a mystery to them. They can't understand why I have so many physical problems. Living with a serious illness is not easy. I've met a lot of sick children; some are in remission, but some died. I thank God that I am still here. I don't feel sorry for myself, because I don't need anyone to feed me, bathe me or dress me. I can do those things for myself. I have one good eye, one good leg and one good arm, which are blessings, because some people don't even have that. I stay encouraged because God is with me, helping me. I've had so many people praying for me and giving me words of encouragement, that it has helped me stay positive. I thank God for all of the doctors and my friends and family, especially my mother. I would like you to read the poem I wrote for her. Her name is Alyce.

MAMA

My mama's name is A.
To some people, she's OK.
But to me she's da world,
A will always be my girl.

She is very nice.
She doesn't shoot dice!
A is very sweet.
She's a person u would love to meet.

She sings a lot of church songs
A tries her best 2 do no wrong.
She is my mama,
And has been there for me
through all the drama.

Happy Mother's Day, Mama

By Kirk, AKA
Da Fster

2014

I graduated with my class in 02. I was able to keep up with my class, thanks to God. I had 2 semesters of accounting at the community college and 2 jobs.

I haven't been to New Orleans in 5 years. I go to the Dr's in Lafayette, La. About 25 minutes from where I live. New Orleans is three hours away. The optometrist is here in Abbeville. My vision is not as good as it used to be. Can't see out of left eye, and the right eye is going to the right.

My next MRI will be in 3 years. The neurosurgery said that it haven't changed since he started seeing me 5 years ago. By the way, I still have that same shunt from Jan. 1989. The endocrinology took me off a few of the med's I was on for a long time. I'm still doing good, and a happy person. Things could be worse for me.

My family is still growing. I have 9 nephews, 8 nieces, and 5 great nephews, 6 great nieces and another nephew due in April 2015. I would like for everyone that will be reading this book to know no matter what happens don't give up on God and yourself. I am 30 years old, blessed with a wonderful family and friends that God put in my life. To help and pray for me. It has not always been easy. But I never gave up on life. I know how to encourage myself. I attend church and a member of the Brotherhood and always take part in the service. My mother is a 2 time breast cancer survivor, and still going strong, and helping out with other family members.

Some things haven't changed, the promises of God are still true. God is still on the throne. The angels are still watching out for God's children, the Holy Spirit is still the Comforter. And Jesus still loves us. Praying that you will be encouraged today.

Love you,

F

Lessons for Adults

Unfortunately, brain tumors are a fact of life: they are the second most common cancer in children, with leukemia being the first. And we don't appreciate that young children can be concerned about them. One study showed that children as young as five who came to their doctors with headaches were worried about having a brain tumor. While our tendency has been to avoid discussing tumors in an effort to protect the children from being frightened, we have to realize that the children are already scared. If the worst happens, they deserve to know the truth.

While the diagnosis of a brain tumor may seem to be the end of the world to us, their parents and doctors, it is just another fact of life to these kids. And sometimes, it appears to be of minor significance. One kid went to New York for surgery, and when she got back, she was hardly interested in the tumor but much more interested in talking about all the things she got to see and do in New York. These kids don't dwell on their disease; perhaps, neither should we.

It was clear that "F" suffered major disabilities as a consequence of either his tumor or the treatment. Yet he did not show any anger because of what he had lost. Instead, he was immensely grateful for what he still had. That is the greatest lesson these kids can teach us.

FINAL LESSONS

(For Adults)

I HOPE YOU HAVE learned as much from these kids as I have. What they want from us adults is remarkably similar, whether they have a tic disorder or juvenile Parkinson's disease. First, they all want to be the ones that are talked to about their disease. One after another, these kids mentioned that they really appreciate it when the doctor talks to them, not just their parents, and they want to be involved in making decisions.

Secondly, all the children in this book stressed that they wanted to know what was wrong with them. I wish I could say I learned this in medical school. Instead, I'm using my own personal experience. When I was thirteen, the doctors thought they saw a tumor on my X-ray and took my father to a separate room to discuss the results. When he returned, he promptly fainted. As you might imagine, I did not believe their reassurances that nothing was wrong. In this book, even Aaron, who received one of the worst diagnoses we could give a child, commented that he wanted to know what was going on. He truly appreciated not being kicked out of the room when the doctor met with the family to give the results of the final testing. The children can all be educated about their problems and how to deal with them. They need to be encouraged to be independent and find solutions to their problems. When possible, I give them the chance to make medical decisions or at least have an input in the discussion. It's nice to see that they, in turn, are eager to teach others. For that was the whole purpose of this book–to allow the children with the condition to teach us and others with the disease.

Finally, none of these children saw themselves as being sick. They consider themselves to be pretty normal kids. They all want to be treated just like everybody else, and their follow-up essays describe adults who have had up and downs in their lives, no different than the rest of us.

CONCLUSION

I HOPE YOU HAVE enjoyed meeting these special kids and reading their stories. We want everybody to understand why their brains work like they do and that you can have these problems and still be a really neat person.

RESOURCES

I HAVE INCLUDED THE addresses of national support groups that can provide a wealth of helpful information and contacts. They will be able to help you get in contact with any local support groups in your area. The contact information is accurate at the time of printing.

Seizures/Epilepsy

Epilepsy Foundation of America
www.epilepsy.com

They have many publications available; some appropriate for children.

Headaches

American Council for Headache Education (ACHE)
www.achenet.org

ADD/ADHD

Attention Deficit Disorder Association (ADDA)
www.add.org

Children with Attention Deficit Disorders (CHADD)
www.chadd.org

Tics / Tourette's Syndrome

Tourette Syndrome Association
www.tsa-usa.org

Autism

Autism Speaks
www.autismspeaks.org

Autism Society of America
www.autism-society.org

Weakness

Families of Spinal Muscular Atrophy (SMA)
www.fsma.org

Muscular Dystrophy Association
www.md.org

Cerebral Palsy

American Academy for Cerebral Palsy and Developmental Medicine
www.aacpdm.org

United Cerebral Palsy Association
www.CerebralPalsy.org

Autoimmune Disorders

GBS/CIDP Foundation
www.gbs-cidp.org

Myasthenia Gravis Foundation of America
www.myasthenia.org

Multiple Sclerosis Association of America
www.mymsaa.org

Brain Tumors

American Brain Tumor Association
www.abta.org

Pediatric Brain Tumor Foundation of the United States
302 Ridgefield Court Asheville, NC, 28806
1-800-253-6530
www.pbtus.org

Pediatric Brain Tumor Foundation
www.curethekids.org

Degenerative Diseases of the Nervous System

National Ataxia Foundation
www.ataxia.org

National Organization for Rare Disorders (NORD)
www.rarediseases.org

Parkinson's Disease Foundation Inc.
www.pdf.org

INDEX

A

ADEM (acute demyelinating encephalomyelitis), 173, 175, 191
ADHD (attention deficit hyperactivity disorder), xiv, 55, 57, 59–62, 64, 66–68, 136, 138–39
Alice in Wonderland (Carroll), 33
Alice in Wonderland syndrome, 33
Asperger's syndrome, 70
attention, 57–58, 60–61, 105, 136, 138
autism, xiv, 55, 69–74, 76, 91–93, 95–97, 102, 105, 212
　classic, 69
autism spectrum disorder, 70

B

behavior, 55, 59, 68, 71, 78, 91, 105, 139
biofeedback, 37
blood, xx, 8, 32, 34–35, 128–29, 138, 147, 176, 179, 192

brain, xvii–xxiii, 5–7, 17–19, 26–27, 31–32, 34–35, 58–61, 109–10, 127–29, 135–38, 141–42, 175–76, 181, 192–98, 214
brain stem, xviii

C

Carroll, Lewis, 33
　Alice in Wonderland, 33
cerebellum, xviii–xix
cerebral palsy, xiv, 107, 109, 127–32, 213
cerebrum, xviii
channelopathy, 120
channels, 120
Charcot-Marie-Tooth disease, 110
chemicals, xviii–xix, 136
chemotherapy, 194
CIDP (chronic inflammatory demyelinating polyneuritis), 173, 175, 213
clubfeet, 114
CSF (cerebral spinal fluid), 176

CT scan (computerized axial
    tomography), xxi, 6–7, 35

D

development, xx–xxi
diseases, autoimmune, 173, 177–78
drugs, 21, 25, 62, 64, 110, 112, 194
dyslexia, 11, 62
dystrophy, 110, 152, 213
    Duchenne muscular, 110

E

EEG (electroencephalogram), xxii, 6,
    12–13, 18, 22, 60, 138
electricity, xviii–xix, xxii, 5, 60, 111–12, 120
EMG (electromyography), xxii, 111–12,
    126
epilepsy, ix, 3, 5–6, 8–11, 21–26, 28–29, 211
exercise, 32

F

Fox, Michael J., 142
Friedreich's ataxia, 141–44

G

gene, xx, 6, 32, 70, 110
Guillain-Barré Syndrome, 110, 173, 175,
    191

H

headache, xiv, 3, 10, 31, 33–41, 45–54,
    84–85, 180, 193, 195–96, 206, 212
    chronic daily, 31, 34–35, 37
    migraine, 10, 35, 44, 47
    muscle contraction, 33
    rebound, 34, 37
    tension, 31, 33–35, 37

heredity, xx–xxi, 39, 70
hyperlexia, 91

I

ibuprofen, 36, 47–48, 53
immune system, 110, 173–75, 183
impulsive, 57, 60
infection, xx, 6–7, 34–35, 70, 173, 183,
    189, 194
insulation, xix
ions, 120

J

Johnson, Samuel, 138
joint position sense, 141

L

lactic acid, 34
leukemia, 34, 206

M

medication, xiv, 17, 22, 43, 53, 62, 68, 74,
    132, 139, 160–61, 165–66, 183
    seizure, 19
    stimulant, 68, 139
medicine, 6–9, 13–14, 21, 23, 26–27,
    33–36, 48–49, 51, 53, 60–65, 78,
    131–32, 176, 178, 185–87
    abortive, 36
    pain, 34
    preventive migraine, 38
    stronger, 36, 53
migraine, xiv, 10–11, 31–40, 42–44, 47,
    53–54
Mozart, Wolfgang Amadeus, 138
MRI (magnetic resonance imaging),
    xxi–xxii, 7, 12, 18, 35, 129, 138,
    147, 176, 181, 185–86, 188, 193,
    197–98, 204

muscles, xiv, xix, xxi–xxiii, 33–34, 37, 109–12, 114, 120–23, 127, 129, 131, 135, 141–42, 146, 175–76
myopathy, 107, 109–10, 126
myotonia congenita, 120–21

N

NCV (nerve conduction velocity), 111, 126
nerve, xiv, xix, xxi–xxiii, 76, 109–12, 114, 116, 120, 127, 135, 141, 145, 175–76
  median, 115, 117–18
nervous system, xiii–xiv, xix, 3, 55, 107, 133, 171, 173, 176, 181, 214
neurologist, xx, xxii–xxiii, 12, 16, 29, 41–42, 45, 47, 50–51, 64, 67, 138, 159–60, 187–88, 197–98
  pediatric, v, 42

O

organ, xix, 8, 192, 197

P

Parkinson's disease, 142–43, 158, 161, 163, 207, 214
pervasive developmental delay, 69
phenobarbital, 21
physician, 29, 105, 191
pill, 8, 36, 42, 132
plasmapheresis, 176, 191
polymyositis, 111
psychologist, 165

S

Sacks, Oliver, 138
sclerosis, multiple, 173, 175, 178, 181, 213
seizure, ix, xiv, xxii, 5–10, 13–21, 23–24, 26–30, 36, 60, 138, 176, 181, 211
  absence, 7–8

focal, 6
  generalized, 6, 21
  generalized tonic-clonic, 8
  grand mal, 6
  partial, 7, 10
side effect, xiv, 8, 53, 60, 68, 138–39
sports, xix, 50, 52, 66–67, 145, 153
status epilepticus, 21
steroids, 176, 183, 187, 189–90, 201
stress, 24, 32, 37, 39, 44, 53, 138–39, 167
stroke, 128

T

test
  blood, xxii, 7, 111, 149, 184, 187
  nerve conduction, xxii
  urine, xxii, 138
therapist
  physical, 112
  speech, 129
therapy
  occupational, 90, 129
  physical, 129
tic, xiv, 55, 60, 135–39, 185, 207, 212
  motor, 135
  vocal, 135
Tourette's syndrome, 55, 60, 136, 138, 212
transverse myelitis, 173, 175, 191
tumor, xx, xxii, 6–7, 34–35, 47, 138, 192–99, 206–7, 214
  brain, xiv–xv, 34–35, 53, 171, 192, 194–96, 198, 206, 214
tumor cells, 193–94

V

vomiting, 50, 53

W

wheelchair, 112, 127, 130, 155–56

www.ingramcontent.com/pod-product-compliance
Lightning Source LLC
Chambersburg PA
CBHW030917180526
45163CB00002B/365